ASTHMA
Stop Suffering, Start Living

SECOND EDITION

M. Eric Gershwin, M.D.

E. L. Klingelhofer, Ph.D.

authors of *Conquering Your Child's Allergies*

W9-BHX-504

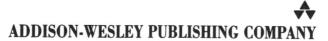

ADDISON-WESLEY PUBLISHING COMPANY

Reading, Massachusetts   Menlo Park, California   New York
Don Mills, Ontario   Wokingham, England   Amsterdam   Bonn
Sydney   Singapore   Tokyo   Madrid   San Juan
Paris   Seoul   Milan   Mexico City   Taipei

Library of Congress Cataloging-in-Publication Data

Gershwin, M. Eric, 1946–
    Asthma : stop suffering, start living / M. Eric Gershwin, E. L.
Klingelhofer. — 2nd ed.
        p.   cm.
    Includes index.
    ISBN 0-201-60847-2
    1. Asthma—Popular works.   I. Klingelhofer, E. L.   II. Title.
RC591.G47   1992
616.2'38—dc20   92-15443
                                                                      CIP

Cover design by Alwyn Velasquez
Text design by Anna Post
Set in 10-point Baskerville by DEKR Corporation, Woburn, MA

Many of the designations used by manufacturers and sellers to distinguish their products are claimed as trademarks. Where those designations appear in this book and Addison-Wesley was aware of a trademark claim, the designations have been printed in initial caps (for example, Adrenalin).

1 2 3 4 5 6 7 8 9-DO-95949392
First printing, September, 1992

Addison-Wesley books are available at special discounts for bulk purchases by corporations, institutions, and other organizations. For more information, please contact:

Special Markets Department
Addison-Wesley Publishing Company
Reading, MA 01867
(617) 944-3700 x 2431

*This is for our wives, Laurel and Jean —
mothers who have dealt with their children's asthma with matchless patience,
resourcefulness, and imperturbability.*

ACKNOWLEDGMENTS

Many hands and minds went into this book. We owe more than we can tell to

- The medical researchers who are gradually unlocking the mysteries of allergy and making it more treatable
- The medical practitioners, upon whose day-to-day experience and wisdom we have drawn heavily
- The American Lung Association chapters and other groups and societies that enthusiastically responded to our requests for information and advice — particularly in compiling the information contained in Chapter 18

We owe special thanks to four people — Samuel Woo, who did the photography, Nikki Rojo, who typed the manuscript and whose energy, intelligence, and matchless skill with the word processor really made the book happen, and Dr. Christopher Chang and Dr. Mark Fletcher, whose meticulous reading of the manuscript caught and eliminated errors of fact and rhetoric.

The mistakes that remain are ours alone.

M. E. G.
E. L. K.

TO OUR READERS

This book can help you and your family greatly. Its suggestions about health care reflect the best and most up-to-date medical information and opinion available. As with all medical advice, however, cases — and therefore treatments — may vary.

The authors and publisher therefore disclaim any responsibility for consequences resulting from following advice or procedures set forth in this book. It is not intended to be an alternative to or substitute for your own doctor's recommendations. In particular, the treatment of severe, protracted, or stubborn symptoms or the use of *any* drug or medication should be undertaken only after consultation with your own physician.

Contents

Introduction to the Second Edition

The six years that have elapsed since the appearance of the first edition of this book have seen profound changes in the ways in which asthma is viewed.

- The underlying nature of the disease has come to be better understood.
- Treatment procedures have been refined and vastly improved.
- New and more effective medications have come into use.
- Regulations governing the availability and use of a number of important triggers have been adopted.

Despite these encouraging developments which have demystified the disease and made it more amenable to treatment, the somber facts are that the incidence of asthma has increased markedly, by more than 30 percent since 1980. Even more alarming are the facts that the number of hospital admissions for its treatment has shot up, and the number of deaths attributed to asthma has nearly doubled since 1976. The reasons for these unsettling trends are complex; certainly degradation of air quality combined with the continuing urbanization of the population is implicated. The increase in the number of poor people and the overrepresentation of children among them has made adequate medical care less readily available for the most vulnerable. Poor or poorly delivered medication bears some share of the blame as well.

Ten million Americans now suffer from asthma. Especially prevalent and troublesome in children, it is a leading cause of absence from school and work. For some people, asthma is just a minor nuisance, only requiring occasional medication; for others, it is a constant, unrelenting struggle for breath. Although asthma is certainly no fun to have or to be around, the good news is that it *can* be controlled.

This second edition of *Asthma; Stop Suffering, Start Living* has been prepared with these realities—positive and negative—firmly in mind. It offers readers the latest information on asthma and strategies they can follow to prevent or control their symptoms. The major objective of this book remains unchanged—to provide the reader with the very latest information about the care of the disease and to impart the skills and attitudes that permit intelligent, aggressive, competent management of it.

This book is a complete, up-to-date, authoritative guide to understanding what asthma is all about—what causes it and how it can be prevented, managed, and treated. The book is solidly founded on scientific knowledge and discoveries—some of them very new. Although it offers no hope of an instant miracle cure, it *will* provide you or your child with the tools you need for a comfortable, normal life.

Our goal is to present the effective use of recent medical treatments, including self-care, in managing asthma symptoms, and to show you how to incorporate other self-help activities to reduce or eliminate your reliance on drugs and devices. Consistent, informed attention to you or your child's illness, coupled with a sound health maintenance program, can make a truly significant difference for you, your family, and your life-style.

We wrote this book out of our genuine desire to help asthmatics. Both of us have had serious problems with asthma in our own families.

Eric Gershwin never planned to be an allergist. What led him to that specialty was his daughter, Tracy, who developed severe asthma as a child. Even so, he probably would not have entered the field if her symptoms had been successfully — or even competently — addressed. The inept, unimaginative, perfunctory care that she received from a succession of physicians led him to conclude that the treatment of asthma and of allergies generally offered him a rare opportunity to provide a real and desperately needed service. He went on to specialize in the field and to devote himself to finding out more about allergic diseases, their causes, and their effective management.

Dr. Gershwin believes that conventional medical procedures are the keystone for successful management of asthma symptoms, but he has also concluded that a comprehensive treatment program that uses aggressive control measures, fosters positive attitudes, and (especially) focuses on prevention is the best approach. He shares this approach with his medical students at the University of California, Davis Medical School, and uses it as the springboard for his diverse research activities.

As a child Ed Klingelhofer had moderate asthma. Every time he caught a cold the infection would go to his chest; he could count on being in bed for three or four days and away from school for a week. This was 60 years and more ago and there wasn't much available then in the way of treatment. If things got really bad the doctor would administer a shot of Adrenalin, which eased the wheezing but made him very hyper and agitated. Because of this reaction to the Adrenalin, the shot was avoided except when it became absolutely necessary, perhaps two or three times a year.

Both of E.K.'s children also had asthma. The older child, a daughter, still does, although she controls it effectively with medications. Her nine-year-old daughter also goes into bronchospasm whenever she catches a cold. His son, as a child, also had moderate asthma, which he outgrew although he shows some wheezing during the pollen season; the son's daughter, now 17, has never shown any signs of the disease.

E.K.'s strongest recollections of those earlier days are of his helplessness, fear, and depression. He sometimes believed that he, and later his children, would never get over the disease, condemned to a lifetime of suffering with many ordinary activities and pleasures denied to them. Even so, they all did everything they could to pursue normal lives, refusing to give in to the disease and trying to do all the things that children and youth do. To a large extent this combativeness kept them from feeling and acting like victims of the disease.

HOW TO USE THIS BOOK

This book is divided into three parts. Part 1 defines and describes asthma. It traces the link between allergies and asthma, outlines the typical course of childhood asthma compared to adult asthma, differentiates asthma from other diseases and conditions, and helps you to diagnose whether or not you have asthma and to determine its cause.

Part 2 discusses various ways to determine what triggers your symptoms, including the role of diet, sports and exercise, chemical and occupational concerns, and allergic complications. Most importantly, it provides you with the precise procedure you will need to follow in order to minimize or avoid what is making you suffer, whether it's how to travel to new places, maintain a special diet, or undergo surgery successfully.

Part 3 looks at the aspects of living with your illness from day to day, including drug therapies, the use of allergy shots, self-help techniques, breathing and other exercises, alternative treatments, and special training and education resources such as summer camps for children.

Naturally you will tend to go directly to the sections that cover the problems or issues that are most puzzling or troubling to you. However, this does not mean that you should pass over the other topics. For instance, if you have asthma you are already familiar with the wheezing, shortness of breath, coughing, and mucus production that are its major symptoms, but do you *really* know what causes your asthma? If your symptoms show up during a cold, do you know why your body reacts the way it does? Understanding the physiological basis for asthma will help you detect and identify what produces or exacerbates your particular symptoms — and how best to treat them.

The most important feature of this book is that it tells you how to approach your illness. Surprisingly, despite all the information and effective medications available today, many asthmatics or their parents still take a passive approach. By doing this they put asthma in charge of their lives, instead of the other way around.

The first step in taking charge of your asthma is to answer the following questions as honestly as possible. If you cannot say yes to each one, look for the motivation and information you need to answer them in this book. It is not always an easy task, and requires effort, diligence, and discipline. But the rewards are vast: a fuller, happier, and healthier life. Good luck!

1. Do you know what asthma is?
2. Do you understand the physiological basis of asthma?
3. Do you know what to expect in an asthma attack?
4. Do you know the early warning signs of an asthma attack?
5. Do you know exactly what medication you are taking and why you are taking it?
6. Do you know where and how to get emergency help if you need it?
7. Have you chosen your doctor carefully?
8. Have you given up smoking?
9. Have you declared your home and workplace a smoke-free zone?
10. Do you follow a regular program of exercise; do you maintain a well-balanced diet?
11. Do you always carry your asthma medications in your pocket or pocketbook?
12. If you are a student, have you told your school authorities that you have asthma?
13. Do you know what foods, drinks, and other triggers to avoid to reduce the chance of an asthmatic attack?

UNDERSTANDING YOUR ASTHMA

What Is Asthma?

WHO HAS ASTHMA?

Asthma may turn up at any age, although it is likely to occur for the first time before the age of five. In childhood it is three times more common and more severe in males, but after puberty the incidence in the sexes is about even. It is more often found in urban, industrialized settings, in colder climates, and among the urban disadvantaged, especially blacks.

Asthma may take many forms, from mild and short-lived exercise-induced wheezing to severe, life-threatening attacks that require emergency hospital treatment. There are few if any ailments that have terrified sick persons and their families more, and more often, than asthma.

Asthma is among the most common of diseases and accounts for more absences from work and school than any other chronic illness. It is a leading cause of visits to the doctor's office. It is a serious disease — the death rate during hospitalization attributed to asthma is under 1 percent in children but rises to 2–4 percent in adults; from 1980 to 1987 the asthma death rate increased by 31 percent.

Individual members of every culture in the world have asthma; there are no areas that are asthma-free. Yet there are striking differences in its incidence and severity among different populations. Presumably these differences are genetic. Asthma is extremely uncommon among West Africans and American Indians. In other parts of the world — Trinidad Island, for instance — 20 to 30 percent of the population has asthma.

Asthma is most common in childhood. Although the predominant feature that determines its presence is inheritance, environment is important. Atopic (allergy-prone) individuals are more likely to be worse if they live on farms with farm animals and crops nearby than if they live in the city. Similarly, there are certain ethnic groups who seem particularly vulnerable. There is an especially high prevalence of severe asthma among African-Americans; black Americans have a much higher rate of hospitalization than white Americans.

Asthma is a serious condition, not to be dismissed as a minor psychological disorder, but it has at least two redeeming features. First, its symptoms are quite likely to become less severe or to vanish altogether as the sufferers grow older. Second, there is a great deal that can be done for asthmatics — or that they can do for themselves — to control, lessen the frequency of, and minimize the severity of their attacks. Furthermore, asthmatics do not, as many authorities mistakenly and carelessly believe, just wheeze or pant their way into old age.

THE SYMPTOMS OF ASTHMA

Asthma (a medical term which originally meant "shortness of breath") is a collection of respiratory symptoms. The most important ones are

- Shortness of breath
- Wheezing
- Coughing
- Increased production of mucus

Shortness of Breath

Shortness of breath (which can develop with amazing rapidity) and wheezing are produced by "twitchy," or spastic, airways. Everybody who suffers with asthma has twitchy air passages. The twitchiness affects the layer of muscle that sheathes the air tubes. In asthmatics this muscle layer is oversensitive; when affected, it contracts, causing the air tubes to constrict. Breathing air, like delivering water through pipes, is more efficiently done through larger tubes.

As air is inhaled it flows through a series of airways. These airways — hollow tubes, really — begin in the throat and descend all the way down to the base of the lungs, branching and proliferating as they go. At the level of the throat and upper chest they are fairly large. The uppermost and largest is called the trachea. About a third of the way down into the chest it branches into two somewhat smaller airways known as main stem bronchi. Each of these main stem bronchi supplies air to one of the lungs.

As the bronchi extend deeper and deeper into the chest, the air tubes divide and proliferate so that they become smaller and smaller. The result is a complex maze of small tubes — airways — which resemble the root structure of a tree (see Figure 1).

The surrounding layer of smooth muscle maintains the size and shape of the airways. When the smooth muscle sheath goes into spasm it chokes or constricts the airways, thus making less room for the air to move in and out of the lung. It is this restriction of air flow that produces the high-pitched wheezing and the struggle to breathe that characterize asthma.

This tendency to twitchiness is usually inherited. In some it is apparent from the moment a child takes its first breath; in others it shows itself on only a handful of occasions during an entire lifetime.

It now seems clear that airway inflammation is the key factor in hyper-responsiveness. However, the tendency for spasm can be made worse by a number of factors. A majority of cigarette smokers, even those unaware of problems with their lungs, have this increased twitchiness of their airways. The twitchiness caused by smoking is in addition to the other lung damage that tobacco wreaks. The most important substances or conditions that aggravate twitchiness are

- Allergies (to foods, pollens, animal dander, etc.)
- Upper respiratory infections of all kinds including ordinary colds
- Cigarette smoking
- Tobacco smoke in a room (secondhand smoke)
- Dust
- A heavy concentration of particles in the air (wood-burning stoves or fireplaces often trigger asthma)
- Exercise or hyperventilation
- Cold air
- Air containing sulfur dioxide, ozone, or smog
- Ingestion of aspirin and the many drugs used to treat arthritis

FIGURE 1   The Respiratory Airways

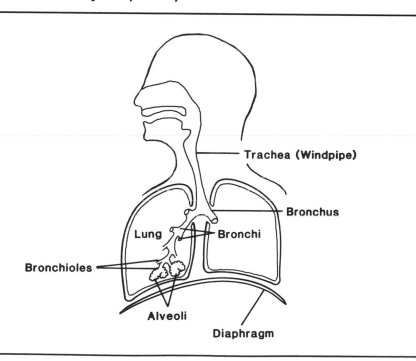

- Certain food dyes
- Foods containing metabisulfite
- Intense emotion, including laughing and crying
- Household or occupational chemicals, vapors, fumes, or dusts
- Nighttime

Most asthmatics know what some of the specific factors that trigger their own asthma are. However, they may be aware of only the major or obvious causes and do not notice minor or incidental contributors. In most people there are several such triggers.

Kevin has had asthma since early childhood. Although he had a rough time when he was younger, the symptoms gradually eased. He still had occasional episodes but could manage them comfortably by avoiding cigarette smoke, dust, and other airborne triggers and by using an Alupent inhaler when he would start to wheeze. He didn't worry much about being asthmatic, though, because he felt he had things under control.

But Kevin was in for a rude awakening. One night he was partying with a few friends and suddenly began to experience serious trouble breathing. He used his Alupent inhaler, but it didn't help; in fact, despite the medication his breathing worsened. Soon he was literally struggling for breath. A friend drove him to the emergency room and there he was given epinephrine and antihistamines. These kicked in quickly and brought relief.

Kevin went to his physician to report the incident and to try to establish its cause. He had not had any symptoms that day and, apart from the partying, had done nothing unusual. No one at the party was a smoker. The doctor asked Kevin if he had eaten anything out of the ordinary that evening. "I had a few glasses of wine and some snacks," Kevin answered.

"What were the snacks?" the doctor asked.

"The usual. Peanuts. Crackers. Cheese. Chips. Salsa."

"Probably something you ate," the doctor said. "Ever have any trouble with any of those things before?"

"Never."

Even though Kevin said he had had no problems with the foods he'd eaten, the doctor instructed him to be careful when he ate those foods in the future. Kevin had a second, milder attack a few weeks after the first one. The circumstances were much the same except that he had eaten only tortilla chips with salsa. Playing a hunch, the doctor asked Kevin to identify the foods' brand names. She then checked the lists of ingredients on the packages. There were no common allergens listed; still, she asked an old friend and colleague at the local medical school to run a series of tests for possible triggers. She found that the salsa, though labeled as fresh, contained an enormous dose of the preservative metabisulfite. The doctor gave Kevin a challenge test with the salsa, and he reacted positively to it. She and Kevin concluded that the sulfite-laced salsa combined with sulfite-laden wine had produced his symptoms.

Kevin's case is typical of individuals suddenly affected by a previously innocuous agent. Although he had eaten foods containing metabisulfite in the past, he had not experienced the massive dose he got from the heavily treated salsa plus the wine.

Wheezing

Most people know what wheezing is, even when they hear it for the first time. It sounds like a breathy whistle or the noise made by an accordion. To test for wheezing, breathe in and out as deeply as you can to clear your throat. Then take a deep breath by inhaling as quickly as you can for as long as you can. Then exhale as fast as you can for as long as you can. While you do this, listen very carefully to the sound you are making. If you do not have asthma all you should hear is the movement of air in and out of your mouth. No sound or noise occurs below the level of the throat. long as you can. Then exhale as fast as you can for as long as you can. While you do this, listen very carefully to the sound you are making. If you do not have asthma all you should hear is the movement of air in and out of your mouth. No sound or noise occurs below the level of the throat. Have someone with asthma do the same maneuver. You will hear a high-pitched, reedy sound if you put your ear against the back of their chest. Sometimes, when people with asthma feel relatively good, you can hear this wheezing only during expiration (breathing out) and only when they exhale quickly and deeply.

It is important to distinguish wheezing from the ordinary sounds associated with breathing. Children with asthma often develop significant swelling and inflammation of their adenoids as well as congestion of nasal passages. These children may seem to snore when they sleep, or their nose may sound squeaky. It is usually easy to distinguish between the noise produced by their nasal obstructions and chest wheezing. Putting your ear to their chest will permit you to make the distinction easily.

Mucus

In addition to the spastic muscle tissue surrounding the airways, mucus-producing cells called *goblet cells* are important contributors to asthma symptoms, particularly the persistent, deep cough. Everybody, asthmatic or not, has these mucus-producing cells.

Mucus is important because it transports the enzymes and chemicals that help the lungs fight infection. Asthmatics have many more of these mucus-producing cells than nonasthmatics, and those with severe asthma have the most goblet cells of all. These cells produce an excess of mucus which clogs airways and obstructs the flow of air, especially in the small airways at the bottom of the lungs.

Mucus is the major lurking problem in asthma. Chronic asthmatics build up large amounts of mucus in their airways. If it is not cleared, it can cause severe breathing difficulties and even death.

THE DIFFERENT TYPES OF ASTHMA

The symptoms of asthma do not vary no matter what is producing them, only their severity. Asthma has so many different causes that it is difficult to catalogue them neatly. One old-fashioned but still useful way to do this is to think of asthma as having three types of causes — extrinsic, intrinsic, and mixed. Your doctor may use one of these words to describe your asthma.

1. *Extrinsic* ("from without") asthma refers to attacks that follow exposure to substances in the environment — dusts, pollens, and the like. It is usually associated with high levels of IgE (immunoglobulin E) and represents a true allergic reaction. Extrinsic asthma, which generally can be reliably diagnosed by skin tests or provoked by challenge tests, ordinarily shows up in childhood, often associated with eczema and hay fever. Curiously, people with extrinsic asthma are also likely to wheeze following exertion or exercise.

Mary's asthma began at about age 8 and lasted until she reached 13. It always showed up in the springtime and was invariably worse on windy days. She began listening to the weather report and soon realized that her symptoms were worse when the pollen count was high. Although Mary's asthma proved difficult to manage during the pollen season, she was symptom-free the rest of the year.

2. *Intrinsic* ("inherent") asthma, found in both children and adults, follows or can be made worse by infection, psychological or emotional stress, and changes in environment or climate. Skin tests are not as useful here, but the typically close correspondence between wheezing and other activities or events makes it easy to spot the cause.

Arthur's asthma began suddenly, eight years ago, when he was 18. It hasn't let up since. He has to take a lot of drugs to remain comfortable and must see his physician several times a year. Although many factors make Arthur's asthma worse, the one thing that always triggers it and makes him extremely sick is viral infection. Arthur was once admitted to the hospital for asthma following a bout of sinusitis and any common cold will send him to the emergency room. Unfortunately, he now has asthma 12 months a year. He went through an extensive battery of allergy skin tests and they were all negative.

3. *Mixed* asthma may have both extrinsic and intrinsic elements.

Jim had eczema in infancy but it went away around age 4. However, at age 6 he began to show signs of hay fever and at age 7 signs of asthma. His asthma, like his hay fever, always came on during the spring and fall. His mother learned to keep the windows closed and kept him indoors on windy days. Jim also wheezed whenever he exercised. As Jim grew older his seasonal symptoms gradually abated. Although they did not vanish, the wheezing was never as bad as it had been when he was in elementary school. However, when he was in his early 20s he began to wheeze when exposed to cigarette smoke and, on occasion, during a cold. Thus, his asthma, which was seasonal in childhood, now occurs year-round and has other factors besides pollen associated with it.

The differences between extrinsic and intrinsic asthma are diagrammed in Figure 2.

WHY ME?

Why me? This is the most common question asthma sufferers ask. The answer is related to certain genetically determined characteristics that may include a predisposition to develop allergies and to have twitchy airways. You can have allergies without asthma, or asthma without allergies. However, the two often go together.

Although more than two-thirds of asthmatics can point to a close family member who has or has had asthma, the complaint is complex and not completely understood. Some individuals from families riddled with asthma never show the disease; others from seemingly clear backgrounds inexplicably turn up with it.

Arthur, the intrinsic asthmatic we discussed earlier, has absolutely no family history of asthma. He is one of seven brothers and three sisters; none of them nor either parent is asthmatic. We do not know why Arthur developed asthma; in Arthur's case the hereditary basis seems not to be a factor.

FIGURE 2   Extrinsic and Intrinsic Asthma

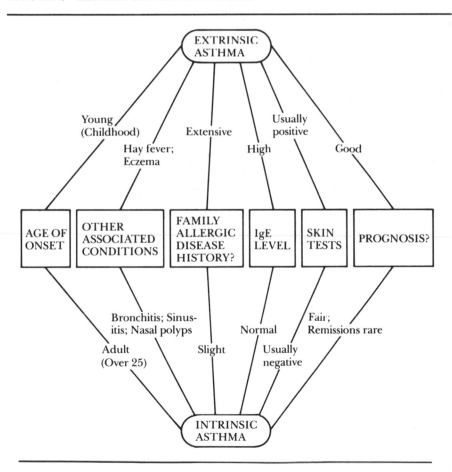

Jim, who has mixed asthma, is an altogether different story. Jim has two brothers and one sister. One brother and one sister have asthma, which started at almost the same age as Jim's. In addition, the asthmatic sister has had severe eczema all her life. Jim's mother has asthma but his father had no allergies whatsoever. Jim's asthma is clearly familial.

In addition to the genes that make you more likely to develop allergies, there may be other genes that determine how severe these allergies may be. However, it is clear that anyone who is *atopic* — genetically disposed to manufacture large amounts of immunoglobulin E (IgE) — is likely to develop allergies to many things. Being atopic is a complex hereditary condition and allergies and asthma are closely tied to it. For a more detailed discussion of allergies and immunoglobulin E, see Chapter 3.

HOW PANIC CAN MAKE ASTHMA WORSE

Because asthmatic symptoms are so obvious and appear to be so life-threatening, sufferers and their families are apt to panic. Panic may intensify the spasms of the airway muscles, which worsens the condition and may impel family members to suggest or supply remedies that only compound the difficulty. Counseling the asthmatic to "breathe deeply and slowly" is a mistake. It causes the asthmatic to hyperventilate, further constricting the airways and worsening the wheezing and shortness of breath. Encouraging coughing does the same thing. It also forces mucus into the airways, blocking them even more. *The acute shortness of breath that defines asthma attacks usually appears to be much more dangerous than it actually is.* If you or someone in your family has asthma, it helps to remember this.

Having asthmatics take tranquilizers (a common and *extremely* dangerous treatment, growing out of the mistaken belief that asthma is due to excitement or emotional upset) only makes things worse. Moreover, severe asthmatics have to keep awake just to breathe harder and more often in order to get the air they need. Sedation — taking tranquilizers — can bring on a sleep that may end in suffocation and death.

ASTHMA LOOK-ALIKES

There are a number of complaints whose symptoms closely resemble those of asthma. These look-alike complaints are not treated the same way as asthma; to mistake them for asthma can be extremely dangerous. That is why a physician's careful differential diagnosis of wheezing and shortness of breath is absolutely essential (see Chapter 13).

Emphysema is a loss in elasticity of the lung tissue brought on, most often, by cigarette smoking or long-time exposure to polluted air. Its external symptoms are shortness of breath, which gets progressively worse, accompanied by a persistent, dry cough. Emphysema hardly ever affects children and is most commonly seen in middle-aged smokers.

> John began to smoke at age 16 and soon developed a pack-a-day habit. At about age 45 he noticed that whenever he got a cold it settled in his chest and seemed to last longer. Still he continued to smoke. At age 50 during what started out as an ordinary cold he became acutely short of breath, turned blue, and collapsed. His wife called the rescue squad, who brought him to the emergency room. John was breathing very rapidly and, while listening to his chest, the emergency room doctor heard some wheezing. John was admitted to the hospital and a chest X ray was done. It revealed a tremendous amount of swelling of the air sacs in his lung. Further studies disclosed that his air tubes were damaged and large air-filled cysts had formed in his lung.

Treatment for emphysema entails respiratory therapy, which may include regular inhalation of oxygen. It is a severely disabling disease and is reaching near-epidemic proportions. Although people with emphysema may wheeze, and although their wheezing is treated much like asthma, the similarity between the two diseases ends there. *Unlike emphysema, asthma is reversible.* Between bouts of symptoms, pulmonary function and airways virtually always return to normal. Moreover, unless there is some infection present, the lung stays intact and, even in the most severe cases, the lung tissue remains normal. Such is not the case in emphysema, where there is actual destruction of the lung itself.

Chronic bronchitis also mimics asthma. Like emphysema, it is frequently found in people who smoke. Workers in certain industries or residents in areas with heavy air pollution often develop bronchitis. For this reason it is more common in large, pollution-plagued cities like Los Angeles.

> Carl has bronchitis. He smoked heavily for about 20 years. He also worked off and on in the coal mines of Pennsylvania. Because of an injury he gave up the mines and moved to be with his daughter in Los Angeles. There he noted that his chronic cough always got worse when he drove on the freeways. When the doctor listened to Carl's chest he sometimes heard wheezing. Unlike people with asthma, though, Carl's bronchitis and cough was always evident. He was never symptom-free. All he can hope for is that his condition will not deteriorate further and that, after flare-ups, he will always return to his borderline status.

Gastroesophageal reflux (GER) is a disease much more common in children than adults. This reflux of the stomach's contents into the esophagus leads to stimulation of the nerves in the esophagus; presumably the nerves precipitate the wheezing. Most patients have symptoms of burping, belching, and heartburn.

> Jimmy, age 3, wakes up every night with wheezing. His mother has frequently complained that he belches a lot. Jimmy's pediatrician recognized that he might have GER and suggested raising the head of his bed 6 to 8 inches. He also told the mother to avoid feeding Jimmy between dinner and bedtime. Jimmy's reflux got much better and his wheezing stopped.

Surgery for GER is possible but is not recommended unless the condition is very severe.

Cystic fibrosis, a tragic disease affecting children, is sometimes mistaken for asthma. Cystic fibrosis runs in families and occurs in both boys and girls. We do not know what produces cystic fibrosis, but we do know that it is characterized by a tremendous increase in the quantity and the thickness of mucus in the airways as well as by an increase in mucus in all body secretions. Even the sweat of cystic fibrosis victims is thicker than that of other people, and sometimes little crystals of salt can be seen to form on their skin. Children with cystic fibrosis experience severe, recurrent bacterial infections which gradually destroy the lung; survival beyond age 20, even with aggressive medical care, is uncommon. These children also often have asthma — so often in fact that, when asthma starts in early childhood, physicians consider the possibility of cystic fibrosis and may order a sweat chloride test to rule out that diagnosis.

> Penny had her first bout of pneumonia when she was only five months old. She was hospitalized, given antibiotics, and recovered without incident. When she was one she was admitted again for pneumonia and recovered. At age 18 months she developed a cold which was accompanied by severe wheezing. That put her in the hospital again. At this point the doctor grew suspicious because Penny had had several episodes of serious respiratory disease in less than two years. He ordered a sweat chloride test and it came back positive. Penny had cystic fibrosis. Even though she had a difficult future, it was extremely important for the doctor to confirm this diagnosis early in her life. It meant that she could have earlier and more aggressive treatment for infections when they occurred.

Foreign objects in the lung can produce asthmalike symptoms. Usually victims of this kind of accident suck in small objects, especially bits of candy or peanuts. However, the variety of foreign bodies doctors pull out of lungs is astonishing — peanuts, M&M's, nails, hair balls, paper clips, seeds, cigarette butts. Even when an object is not picked up by X ray, the affected lung will show inflammation. Or the doctor's exam will disclose that the wheezing is confined to only one lung. Foreign-body wheezes in only one lung are not due to asthma.

> Six-year-old Robin ate too many peanuts. She felt fine, but after three or four days her mother (who did not know about the peanuts) noted that she was coughing and her skin seemed a little blue. She also had a wheeze. Robin was taken to her doctor, who listened to her chest and thought she could have asthma. Still, it didn't sound quite right. To be on the safe side he ordered an X ray. The X ray showed that the lung had collapsed in one of the lobes on her left side. This suggested an obstruction in the airways. He hospitalized Robin and had a pediatric chest specialist examine her. The chest specialist did a bronchoscopy (inserted a long, flexible tube into her mouth and down her windpipe) and in the process saw and was able to retrieve the peanut without an operation.

The Onset and Course of Asthmatic Disease

ASTHMA AND AGE

The intrinsic and extrinsic causes of asthma we discussed in Chapter 1 are tied to age. Furthermore, asthma can occur with or without the presence of the hereditary allergic mechanism IgE. As we mentioned in Chapter 1, IgE-caused asthma is called atopic. (We discuss IgE more fully in Chapter 3.)

If first attack occurs	then	*the likely cause is*
before age 5		non-atopic (intrinsic asthma)
from 5 to 20		atopic (allergy-caused; IgE-linked or extrinsic asthma)
over 20		non-atopic (intrinsic asthma)

Whether the cause is related to allergies or not, all asthmatics have and owe their symptoms to twitchy airways which can be pushed into spasm by exercise, emotion, infection, irritants, or medications. The susceptibility of airways to spasm depends on age. Younger individuals are more vulnerable; however, the environment makes its own important contribution to the onset and severity of asthmatic attacks. Regardless of age, though, a one-time asthmatic has airways that, under certain conditions, can react again.

THE COURSE OF CHILDHOOD ASTHMA

Sean was an obliging, cheerful, fun baby. Then, just before his second birthday, he came down with a cold, and his parents noticed that he was having trouble with his breathing. They took Sean to the doctor and she prescribed some medications that relieved the cold, and the breathing problem went away. However, both parents had had allergy problems when they were children and they rightly feared the worst.

Thereafter, every time Sean had a cold it would slip into an asthma attack, and the attacks kept getting worse and worse. Finally, at the onset of even the slightest sniffle, the parents knew that there would come a time when they would have to rush him to the emergency room for epinephrine (Adrenalin) injections. Without those injections he would struggle for each breath, his color gradually changing, his lips going blue as his body got less and less of the oxygen it needed. His parents were filled with dread. They were frightened and felt helpless.

Then Sean started wheezing even when he didn't have a cold. His mother noticed that his wheezing coincided with her ragweed-induced attacks of hay fever. She mentioned it to the doctor, who agreed that the ragweed was probably making matters worse.

The family talked things over and decided to move to a part of the country that was ragweed free. They were fortunate in that the father, a salesman, could transfer to another office of the company he worked for. They chose Nevada, where Sean's and the mother's ragweed allergies disappeared immediately. Sean's attacks of asthma continued for a time whenever he had a cold but became milder and milder as he grew older. He had his last severe attack when he was 7 and his last attack ever when he was 10. Now an adult, he is largely free of symptoms, although he does wheeze a little, coughs, and produces a lot of mucus whenever he mows the lawn and disturbs one of the large, pollen-dusted rice-paper plants which line the patio. He also wheezes slightly following vigorous exercise.

Asthma is most common in children. There is a good reason for this; asthma affects smaller airways more drastically than larger ones. When larger airways collapse there is still enough room for air to move, but when small airways constrict they may completely block the passage of air. In children, especially children under six, more than 80 percent of the airways are anatomically small. From the age of six and progressively thereafter the percentage of small airways decreases until it reaches 20 percent. For that simple reason asthma is always worse, and most frightening, in very small children.

During early childhood more boys than girls have asthma. As they get older, boys are more likely to show improvement, so that by puberty (12–13 years) the numbers of boys and girls with asthma are nearly equal.

"He (or she) will outgrow it," parents often hear. This is not entirely accurate. Childhood asthma gets better as the lung anatomy changes to contain a larger percentage of bigger airways. Because most children have mild asthma they become relatively free of visible symptoms as they grow older. Yet, they still have twitchy airways, and if they are subjected to enough of the aggravating factors we listed at the beginning of Chapter 1 they may once again start wheezing. This can happen when they are considerably older — even when they are adults.

The twitchiness, or hyperirritability, of the airways also eases with age for reasons that are unclear, but it may have something to do with the maturing of the smooth muscle that overlies the airways.

Henry had his first asthma attack when he was three years old; later episodes caused major problems in the family. Henry's father thought the asthma was due to emotional causes and could be prevented if Henry were "strong" and "mature" and would "grow up." Henry's mother thought of him as an invalid who needed to be protected and sheltered from everything in sight. This disagreement produced some fine arguments.

Despite his misguided parents, Henry improved as he got older, and by the time he was 12 he was largely free of symptoms, even when he forgot to take his medication. Naturally his mother was gratified that her protectiveness had worked; the father was glad that the kid had finally grown up.

Henry went on to college and then to medical school. One of his lecturers, an allergist, said that children do not outgrow asthma and that if they were properly challenged they would have a tendency to wheeze.

Henry disagreed. "I was an asthmatic once," he said, "but I don't have it any more."

"That's what you think," the lecturer said. "You've still got it. You just don't know it."

They went off to the pulmonary function clinic in the hospital. Henry was surprised to discover that when his air flow was measured it was slightly reduced. Worse, after a 15-minute session on a treadmill, even though he felt fine, further measurements showed even more reduction in air flow and a slight tendency to wheezing.

"You've still got it," the allergist said. "It's just not a problem any more."

Henry agreed grudgingly. He didn't mention it to his parents.

One should not conclude that, because the symptoms have gone away, the asthmatic predisposition has gone with them. Older individuals who had childhood asthma and who are stressed by exercise or who inhale certain irritant materials often learn that the asthmatic tendency persists. Sometimes frequency and severity of symptoms decline in individuals who, when they were young, had wheezed following viral infections. Their asthma gets better as they grow older, but this is partly because the number of viral infections we are subject to decreases as we age. A child of two may have as many as 10 to 15 colds a year; a 12-year-old, on the other hand, usually has only three or four colds a year. In short, we develop immunity to many of these infections, and the asthma attacks and the colds decrease together. In fact, some of these asthma-triggering infections, such as respiratory syncytial virus infection — a condition caused by syncytium, a complex form of virus — are much more prevalent in very young children. If you tend to wheeze primarily as a result of respiratory infection, your asthma will likely improve either as the cold season passes or as the number of colds diminishes.

However, as you get older you may also begin to wheeze for other reasons. For example, beginning about age 5, allergies may cause increased twitchiness. Whether the asthmatic child becomes predisposed by viral infections to develop allergies or is merely experiencing a different manifestation of the same underlying cause, namely spastic or twitchy airways, is a question still being argued by medical researchers. It is clear that if you had respiratory virus–induced asthma as an infant you have about a 50 percent chance of continuing to have asthma as you get older.

Fortunately, though, you as a worried parent of a wheezing and asthmatic child can expect that your and your child's life will become considerably easier as he or she gets older. Even so, try not to forget that your child has asthma. This information may be helpful when your child becomes older and faces challenges that may trigger an underlying genetic predisposition.

There are many examples of famous asthmatics — including those who lived long before the advent of modern medical therapy — who have overcome the problems of their asthma to lead vigorous adult lives. Perhaps the best known is Teddy Roosevelt. Teddy suffered his entire life from severe asthma. He was frequently hospitalized, often bedridden, had a severe chronic cough, and had difficulty raising mucus and other secretions. As a child he was unable to keep up with his peers, was considered sickly, and thought unlikely to survive to adulthood. However, he was a determined individual who, with the help and encouragement of his father, pushed himself. The strenuous exercises that he did increased his respiratory capacity and helped reduce the frequency and severity of his attacks. Although his wheezing continued throughout his life, it never interfered with his activities as big game hunter, soldier, president, and conservationist.

Myths about Childhood Asthma

There are so many misconceptions and so much folklore about asthma in children that it is important to remember the following:

- Emotional disorders *do not* cause asthma. Rather, having asthma can precipitate emotional problems.
- Children with asthma *can* and *should* participate in sports and athletic activities. They *can* play musical instruments; in fact, playing wind instruments is beneficial and builds up respiratory muscle reserve.
- Asthmatic children *can* grow up and pursue any type of career or hobby, *providing* their asthma is adequately controlled and their work environment or activities are free of triggers for wheezing.
- Children with asthma *can* safely undergo surgery.
- Asthma *does not* cause emphysema. It *does not* destroy the lung and it is a totally reversible process. Between attacks of asthma the lungs are completely normal.

- Children with asthma *should* experience normal growth and *will not* develop chest deformities. Only if they are given medications like cortisone will this occur, and then only rarely.
- Asthmatic children *can* attend birthday and slumber parties; sleeping bags and pillows cause attacks only when they contain a trigger or allergen. Candles on birthday cakes are a problem only when the smoke is inhaled.
- Asthmatic children should *not* be sent to special care facilities unless their asthma is extremely difficult to control and requires constant direct medical attention.
- *No one* who has had asthma in adolescence is eligible for military service.
- If your first child has asthma, it *does not* necessarily mean that a second will also be asthmatic.
- Most asthmatic children *will* significantly improve by following a regular program of medication.
- Tonsillectomy and adenoidectomy *do not* cure asthma and should *not* be done simply for asthma.
- Wheezing is *not* found in every child with asthma. Sometimes a persistent cough may be the only symptom.

THE USUAL COURSE
OF ADULT-ONSET ASTHMA

Ernie has lived in San Francisco all of his life and had never been troubled by allergies. However, he recently bought a house and a few months after he moved into it he began to cough at night. The cough kept getting worse and attacks of wheezing began.

Things eventually got so bad that Ernie consulted an allergist who put him through a series of skin tests. They showed Ernie as having sensitivity to cat dander. The allergist asked if the previous owners had had pets.

Ernie checked with the previous owners and learned that they had kept three cats, all long hairs, and all of them house cats. Even though he had vacuumed the place thoroughly and redecorated before moving in, the wall-to-wall carpets were full of animal dander.

Ernie had the shag carpeting removed and replaced with new low-pile nylon carpeting after cleaning and vacuuming the bare floors carefully. He also had the drapes dry-cleaned.

His wheezing stopped immediately, but it started coming back under extremely windy weather conditions or sometimes when Ernie caught a cold. It also flared up again when his girlfriend got a kitten.

Adult asthma is more apt to crop up abruptly following environmental or climatic changes that are substantial enough to trigger latent sensitivities. Symptoms may appear at home or, frequently, as a result of materials encountered in the workplace. The causes of adult asthma are often difficult to track down. One big problem with adult-onset asthma is that it does not go away, and unfailing avoidance tactics and scrupulous preventive measures need to be taken to ward off attacks.

WHY YOU SHOULD PAY ATTENTION TO YOUR (OR YOUR CHILD'S) ASTHMA

Asthma must be taken *seriously*. It is simply not true that asthmatics just wheeze their way into old age. Despite the fact that asthma is easily managed, you should not assume that during a given episode you will not need medication.

Judy had severe asthma during infancy. Her symptoms most often started with a cold. As she got older, her wheezing decreased and she found she needed medication only occasionally. During adolescence she had no problems at all with her asthma other than some mild wheezing during gym class. She generally carried around a metered aerosol of Ventolin with her but hardly ever used it. Then Judy went on a class trip and visited a shop that manufactured candles. The strong odor from the candle shop made Judy begin to cough. She suddenly found the coughing was making her wheeze and she could not catch her breath. She went outside, thinking to get her Ventolin out of her handbag. She scrabbled around and suddenly realized that she was no longer carrying any. The only Ventolin she had was four years old and buried somewhere in her dresser drawer. Judy's wheezing became severe and, while the rest of her classmates went on with their outing, she was rushed to a hospital emergency room where she received injections of Adrenalin and some oxygen until her acute symptoms abated.

Although it pays to be prepared for an asthmatic emergency — even if you have not had one in years — you should not think that you are an invalid, sentenced to a life of suffering just because you are an asthmatic. There are millions of fellow sufferers out there. Be prepared. Do not be ashamed or embarrassed to carry your metered aerosol or your medications on airplanes, in foreign countries, or on visits to the homes of family or friends. It is far less embarrassing to use a metered aerosol quietly than to have a full-blown emergency because you aren't carrying medication to treat yourself.

Allergies and Asthma

The word *allergy* conjures up a host of meanings. To those of us who suffer from them, allergies can be anything from a minor nuisance to a frightening, ever-present threat to life. The causes are not as well understood as those of most other medical conditions and so treatment sometimes appears to be little more than educated guesswork.

To many, the word *allergy* seems strange and exotic, which may help to explain its careless and widespread application. It has even taken on nonmedical connotations: "Maybe I'm allergic to my desk," states Peppermint Patty, the cartoon strip character, to explain her poor grades.

Those fortunate enough to be free of allergies are inclined to regard an allergic person as a mystery, a crank, a hypochondriac, a malingerer, or a pitiable weakling. They have little understanding of the misery wrought by allergies and cannot sympathize with the millions who suffer from a staggering variety of allergic complaints. They cannot fully comprehend the anxiety and dread of a mother who does not know the cause of her child's allergy or even if allergy is involved; the acute discomfort and self-consciousness of an adult who endures hives and chronic itching; the agony of a teenager trying to live through the maddening discomfort and disfigurement of persistent eczema; the sense of failure experienced by a student with severe hay fever whose grades suffer because of the sedation produced by antihistamines.

Even people who treat allergies have wide-ranging views of what an allergy is. To the more medically conservative practitioner it is a specific set of conditions verified by rigorous laboratory tests. To others it is any of a broad and ill-defined series of reactions that almost everyone has at one time or another.

Medical authorities generally use the word *allergy* to refer to the hypersensitivity of the body to a specific substance, usually termed an *allergen* or *antigen*, that results in any of a wide variety of reactions. Some allergic reactions are eczema, hives, hay fever, vascular problems — and, most important to us here, the wheezing, shortness of breath, and mucus production that attend asthmatic attacks.

Your asthma is more than likely to be the result of, or at least made worse by, allergies. Out of a population of roughly 250 million in the United States, an estimated 37 million (15 percent) have some sort of allergic disease; about 10 million (4 percent of the total population and over 25 percent of all allergy sufferers) have asthma.

WHAT IS AN ALLERGY?

Many authorities believe allergies originated millennia ago with the human body's evolution of mechanisms to rid itself of invading worms and parasites. The body fights these invaders by producing a special antibody called immunoglobulin E — IgE, for short. This antibody, a chemical released into the blood, helps the body attack and destroy foreign materials, especially those in the gut or lung.

Most parasites enter and live either in the lung or in the intestines of the host. Lining the interior surface of the lung and the intestine are special groups of lymph nodes. These lymphoid tissues harbor the cells that have the machinery to make IgE.

The production of IgE was once perhaps essential to man's attempt to survive the threat of parasites. However, as civilization (and hygiene) advanced, the prevalence of human parasites declined and the need to fight worms with IgE became less important. For most of us in the Western world, these special IgE-producing cells are no longer needed.

Nonetheless, these redundant cells continue to exist, and, although they are not ordinarily called on to fight parasites, they continue to react to the presence of other foreign substances in the body. And, because they are found in the lung and the gut, they are among the first tissues to encounter those things that enter the body from the outside world; they monitor everything inhaled and eaten. Some people have a predisposition, probably inherited, to manufacture large quantities of IgE. This higher level of IgE does no apparent good; worse, it is associated with most forms of allergic disease. Individuals with this genetic tendency are often called *atopic*, a word that connotes people with allergies.

Allergy, then, is nothing more than a reflection of the individual's production of this special antibody known as IgE. Those who make lots of it generally have allergies; everyone else has levels that are either irrelevant or too low to provoke an allergic reaction. Accurate diagnosis and efficient management of allergic symptoms rest on the detection and measurement of IgE.

WHAT HAPPENS IN THE BODY
TO TRIGGER AN ALLERGIC REACTION?

Most of the air we breathe and the food we swallow contain pollens and chemicals considered foreign by the body. Our bodies process these foreign materials in one of two ways — either by routinely processing and degrading the allergen or antigen and excreting it or by degrading the antigen but also producing IgE to react against it. Production of IgE appears to be an attempt to accelerate the elimination of the allergen. Unfortunately, the process of manufacturing this antibody also activates an entire new battery of body immune machinery.

The process is easy to understand. The IgE antibody that is produced binds onto certain white blood cells in the body. These white cells are known as mast cells and basophils. The IgE antibodies are constantly on guard, like a sentry, looking out for foreign bodies or chemicals (allergens) while attached to these white cells. If the allergen enters the body, as when a grass pollen is inhaled or a particular food eaten, it is quickly detected by these sentry IgE antibodies. The sentries, as soon as the allergen touches them, shoot holes in the white cells. The white cells, because they now have holes in their walls, release stored chemicals, the most important of which is histamine. It is the release of this histamine and the other stored chemicals that causes allergic symptoms such as flushing, wheezing, and hives. Unhappily, the white cells are not content to stop at that point. Once the sentry has made the holes, the white cells begin to synthesize a whole new group of chemicals in the body. Some of these chemicals include substances known as prostaglandins and leukotrienes. These materials may require from several hours to as long as several days to be produced by the white cells. However, once they are manufactured and released, they may cause persistent, severe, and stubborn allergic symptoms. Thus, the elements that combine to produce allergic symptoms include the presence of the allergen (a substance you are allergic to), the IgE antibodies, and the white cells.

THE DANGER OF ALLERGIES

Sometimes it is impossible to predict the severity of an allergic reaction. For example, two young men, each 18 years of age, may see the same doctor for a strep throat. Each has received penicillin many times before. Both are given the same prescription for penicillin. One takes the penicillin for 10 days, clears the strep infection, and goes his merry way. The other takes the penicillin and, within a few minutes of swallowing the first pill, breaks out in hives, begins to wheeze, has acute shortness of breath, and experiences a serious drop in blood pressure. Without immediate emergency treatment this man could die.

Fortunately, of the millions of Americans who suffer from allergies, most experience only minor inconveniences. They are troubled by hay fever during the pollen season, or they may have an occasional bout of hives or eczema as a child. For most of these individuals antihistamines purchased over-the-counter, coupled with an occasional visit to a physician, enable them to manage their symptoms comfortably.

HOW REPEATED EXPOSURE MAKES ALLERGIES WORSE

It is common practice in childhood to immunize against diphtheria, whooping cough, tetanus, polio, and measles. These vaccinations are extremely effective.

The process of immunization usually involves a series of injections, or shots. Pediatricians know that there are certain ages and intervals between shots that make immunization most effective. For example, a child may require several doses of a polio virus before developing adequate immunity. With each dose of the vaccine the body makes a better and better antibody response. This process is known as sensitization; and, when the child is adequately sensitized, sufficient antibodies are on hand to fight off the disease.

This same process of sensitization is also required for the appearance of IgE antibodies. The body must encounter allergens over a long enough period of time before they set off an adequate IgE response. Many people have to be exposed to an allergen scores of times before even small amounts of IgE are seen. To people who are known as atopic, IgE antibodies may show up after brief or casual exposure.

Jack, a 43-year-old carpenter, had lived in New York City all of his life and had hardly ever ventured out into the country. Jack had been essentially healthy and had never suffered from any allergies. For business reasons he moved to Sacramento, California, sometimes called the Queen City of Allergies.

The first year he resided in Sacramento Jack's health remained good. The second year he began to experience some springtime hay fever. The third year, however, Jack developed severe hay fever, chronic sneezing, and itchy red eyes in springtime. For the next several years spring meant suffering for Jack. He finally made the allergy connection one May when he left the Sacramento area to visit his family in New York. Within a few days of arriving in New York his symptoms abated. Jack's business was doing well in Sacramento so he returned there, although he now requires the care of an allergist to hold his symptoms to manageable levels.

Jack had the predisposition to develop allergies all along but needed two years of exposure to the pollens in Sacramento for his symptoms to appear. He did not have hay fever in New York because New York is not as rich an agricultural area as is Sacramento and has fewer and different pollens.

> Dr. Pierce is an oral surgeon. He is an active jogger who stays in good shape. He neither smokes nor drinks. During childhood he suffered from scarlet fever and was given an injection of penicillin. The scarlet fever improved, but he remembers that for several weeks after the injection he had hives. It has been more than 20 years since the scarlet fever, and Dr. Pierce has not had to take penicillin since. One morning he wakes up with a severe sore throat. His doctor diagnoses a strep infection. Accordingly he gives Dr. Pierce a prescription for penicillin. Dr. Pierce reminds the family physician of the hives he suffered from as a child. The physician is rightly concerned that Dr. Pierce might be allergic to penicillin and prescribes an antibiotic known as Keflex. Dr. Pierce takes the Keflex and within minutes collapses in his study wheezing and desperately short of breath — an anaphylactic shock reaction. He is rushed to the emergency room and immediately given an injection of Adrenalin and recovers without incident. Dr. Pierce is in fact allergic to penicillin; his family doctor forgot that a small percentage of patients who are allergic to penicillin also have a cross-reactivity to other antibiotics, among them Keflex.

It is important to know not only what you are allergic to but whether there are other substances that share enough characteristics with the offender to produce a cross-reaction. Peaches, for example, are in the same food family as almonds. If you are allergic to peaches you are also likely to be allergic to almonds. (See Appendix E.)

If a person lives in the same area for a long time, the sensitization process occurs with every season. And, as the seasons roll around, the amount of IgE produced by the atopic person may go up and up. In fact, if you measure the quantity of IgE in the blood of a hay fever sufferer regularly over a period of 12 months, you will find that the level rises with the onset of the pollen season and is often at its lowest before the beginning of the next season.

One common treatment for allergies — perhaps the most popular medically administered one — is to deliver injections that introduce the offending antigen into the body in a series of gradually increasing dosages. This procedure, if appropriate for your condition, and if it works, often succeeds in desensitizing you to the offending substance. In effect, it modifies the process by which your allergy established itself in the first place. For further discussion of common allergies associated with asthma, see Chapter 4; Chapter 16 reviews the use of allergy shots.

4.

Allergic Complications Associated with Asthma

Asthmatics whose symptoms are the result of an allergic reaction (you remember that these people are called *atopic*) are prone to develop a number of other troublesome medical problems as well.

ECZEMA

Eczema (*atopic dermatitis,* or AD) is the most tenacious and disturbing of the allergic skin disorders. It usually shows up between the second and sixth months of life and may persist for years or, rarely, for an entire lifetime. It affects about 4 children in 100 and is somewhat more prevalent among females; it is more likely to be encountered in urban and industrialized areas; and it plays no ethnic or racial favorites.

The most prominent feature of eczema is the intense itching it provokes, an itch so maddening that scratching becomes irresistible and brings on the ugly and disfiguring sores that are the hallmark of the disorder. It is often referred to as "the itch that rashes."

> Charles had a severe case of eczema, which the doctor suspected he was making worse by scratching, even though Charles denied this vehemently. He permitted the doctor to put a plaster cast over his lesions, then went home and scratched right through the cast. The same doctor treated Paul in the same way. Paul was able to keep from scratching and when the cast was removed the skin was clear.

Whether or not a skin disorder is eczema can be determined by consulting the decision chart illustrated in Figure 3. However, the character and location of the disorder varies with the age of the victim: *infant* eczema

FIGURE 3   Decision Chart for Eczema

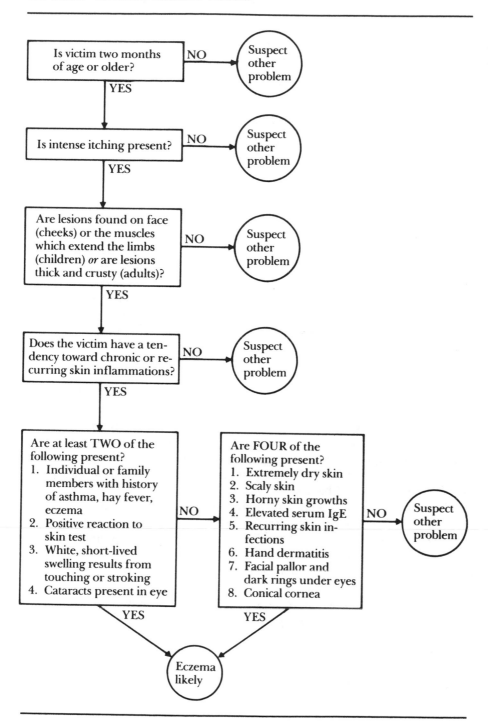

starts after the second month, and most sufferers are clear of symptoms by the second year. The "moist" or "wet" type is most common at this stage; the face, and especially the cheeks, of the baby are the favorite sites for the lesions. *Childhood* eczema shows up after the second year and is usually gone by the 10th birthday. Generally these children have "dry" eczema, which characteristically shows scaling. Distinct, flat, dry elevations on the skin predominate; lesions are most often found at the insides of the elbows and knees, on the neck, and on the skin behind the ears. *Adolescent* and *adult* eczema appear at adolescence or later. The "dry" type of lesion is prevalent in this stage, often confined to the hands.

The cause or causes of eczema remain a mystery. Its sufferers, when tested in the laboratory, sometimes show elevated levels of specific immunoglobulin E, and there is a very strong likelihood that individuals with eczema will display asthma or hay fever symptoms as well. Parents and physicians have observed that the condition may break out or grow worse during peak pollen seasons or after eating certain foods.

Carefully conducted experiments using skin tests that tried to tie hypersensitivity to specific foods to eczema have proved inconclusive. In any case, routine skin testing for individuals suffering from eczema is not recommended because of the risk of triggering a reaction or worsening an existing one. Thus, all that can be said about eczema symptoms is that they are associated or linked with other bodily signs and are quite possibly made worse by exposure to allergy-producing substances to which the individual is susceptible — foods, dust and pollens, animal dander, molds. Consequently the sufferers or their parents must rely on elimination diets (see Appendix A) or careful, critical observations to identify the agents that appear to produce or worsen the symptoms. *Because of the possible role of foods in producing eczema, newborn children with allergic parents should be breast-fed for at least their first six months.* This will delay the need to feed babies formula, cow's milk, and other foods until later in the first year of life. Breast-fed babies have less eczema (indeed, fewer allergies of *all* kinds) than bottle-fed babies.

The treatment of eczema has to take into account a number of factors — type and extent of the disease, age and occupation of the victim, presence or absence of infection. Figure 4 sketches the steps and strategies for home treatment of eczema.

To the eczema sufferer, the most disturbing features are the unbearable itching, the unsightliness of the lesions, and how others view them. It is almost impossible to keep from scratching, an impulse that may have caused the lesions in the first place, may make them worse, or may even bring on a secondary infection. In Figure 4 are listed various means of overcoming this powerful urge to scratch; controlling it is vital to the successful treatment of allergic skin disorders. These methods, if they are given a chance and if they are backed up by a determination not to scratch, will work.

Because society places a high value on clear skin, the unsightly lesions often set in motion a chain of events that only makes a bad situation worse.

FIGURE 4 First Aid and Home Treatment for Eczema

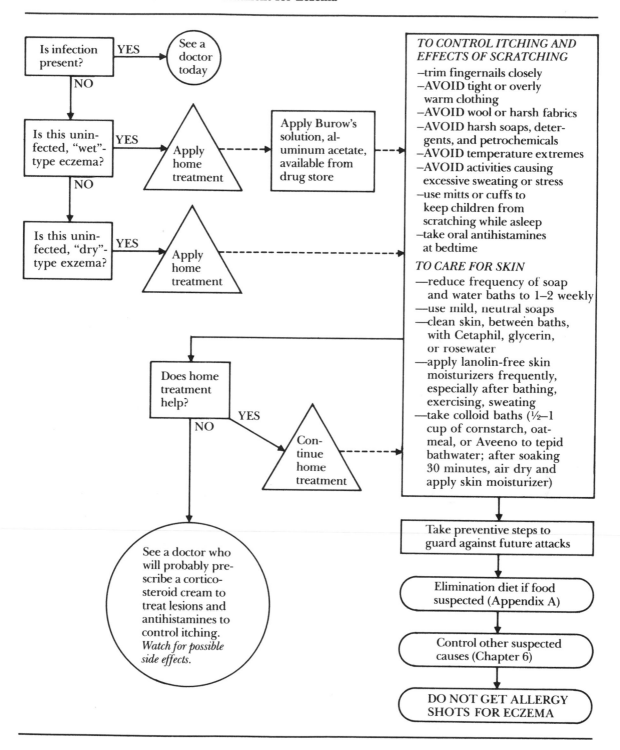

Is infection present? —YES→ See a doctor today

Is infection present? —NO→

Is this uninfected, "wet"-type eczema? —YES→ Apply home treatment ----→ Apply Burow's solution, aluminum acetate, available from drug store ----→

Is this uninfected, "wet"-type eczema? —NO→

Is this uninfected, "dry"-type exzema? —YES→ Apply home treatment ----→

TO CONTROL ITCHING AND EFFECTS OF SCRATCHING
–trim fingernails closely
–AVOID tight or overly warm clothing
–AVOID wool or harsh fabrics
–AVOID harsh soaps, detergents, and petrochemicals
–AVOID temperature extremes
–AVOID activities causing excessive sweating or stress
–use mitts or cuffs to keep children from scratching while asleep
–take oral antihistamines at bedtime

TO CARE FOR SKIN
—reduce frequency of soap and water baths to 1–2 weekly
—use mild, neutral soaps
—clean skin, between baths, with Cetaphil, glycerin, or rosewater
—apply lanolin-free skin moisturizers frequently, especially after bathing, exercising, sweating
—take colloid baths (½–1 cup of cornstarch, oatmeal, or Aveeno to tepid bathwater; after soaking 30 minutes, air dry and apply skin moisturizer)

Does home treatment help? —YES→ Continue home treatment ----→

Does home treatment help? —NO→ See a doctor who will probably prescribe a corticosteroid cream to treat lesions and antihistamines to control itching. *Watch for possible side effects.*

Take preventive steps to guard against future attacks

Elimination diet if food suspected (Appendix A)

Control other suspected causes (Chapter 6)

DO NOT GET ALLERGY SHOTS FOR ECZEMA

Most eczemas are eventually controlled and leave no scars; however, the temptation to disguise or mask the lesions with cosmetics often proves irresistible. This compounds the problem because many cosmetics are in themselves allergens and can intensify the symptoms; scratching introduces the cosmetic into the lesion and this invasion quickly makes matters worse. Moreover, consumers often choose beauty preparations on the strength of what their manufacturers say about their properties; these claims can be misleading. For instance, so-called gentle Ivory is considered to be harsh and irritating by many medical authorities and should be scrupulously avoided by anyone with eczema. After weighing the trivial advantages of a cosmetic cover-up against the potential risks, we strongly counsel patience and a small measure of self-denial.

The support and understanding of others is especially important to the treatment of eczema, since anxiety and stress are a component of and a known contributor to these complaints. Friends and family can help if they realize the following:

- Apart from the skin disorder, the sufferer (unless troubled with asthma or hay fever) is in excellent health.
- The condition can be diagnosed, cured, or controlled and will have no serious aftereffects — even though the allergist may not be able to determine the underlying cause.
- Allergic skin disorders are *not* transmitted from person to person — that is, people who have them can handle food and socialize freely with *no* danger of transmitting their complaint to others.
- Allergic skin disorders are not the fault of those who have them.

Once one understands eczema, other actions can be taken to aid and support the sufferer:

- Work toward a stress-free environment that avoids criticism, nagging, picking on, harping at, or making fun of the sufferer.
- Hold conferences with the doctor and within the family to bring about a full understanding of the nature of the disorder, to plan management steps, to determine whose responsibility they are, and to show how others can help see they are carried out.
- Locate other victims of the same disorder and aid the sufferer to get in contact with them. This step can be done by or aided by hospital or doctor. In some places throughout the country support groups ("eczema clubs," for example) have been formed to help sufferers and their families.

HAY FEVER

Almost 25 million Americans have hay fever (allergic rhinitis) with or without asthma. Next to dandruff it is probably America's most common chronic condition.

When associated with asthma and eczema, hay fever is extremely likely to be atopic or allergic in origin. Perhaps 5 million Americans suffer from this particular combination of problems. In them hay fever is more accurately termed allergic rhinitis.

Allergic rhinitis can be triggered by an astonishingly long and diffuse list of substances that are inhaled — house dust, molds, pollens, insect parts, animal dander, and, increasingly often nowadays, airborne chemicals and irritants encountered in the workplace. Plant products, vegetable gums (present in denture adhesives and tooth powders), insecticides, hair sprays, and many other inhaled substances have all been found to cause "hay" fever.

Hay fever differs from asthma and eczema, the other two members of the allergic triad, in a number of ways. It is likely to show up somewhat later in life, after sensitization has occurred; it generally does not clear up or remit as you grow older; and it is often comfortably and safely controlled with shots. Fortunately, hay fever is usually mild and seasonal, and, for most sufferers, represents nothing more than a brief period of discomfort, which can be managed quite effectively with over-the-counter antihistamines.

The symptoms of hay fever are so well known that they almost need no description or elaboration. They include:

1. Recurrent sneezing, often 5 to 10 times consecutively; worse in the morning
2. Itchy, smarting, watery eyes
3. An "itch" in the roof of the mouth, ear canals, or throat (you want to "scratch" your throat with your tongue)
4. Allergic "shiners," or circles under the eyes
5. Chronic mucus discharge from the nose
6. Chronic nasal stuffiness, often compelling mouth-breathing
7. Wrinkling and scratching your nose
8. Rubbing your nose, particularly in an upward direction
9. Unexplained nose bleeds
10. Loss of the sense of taste or smell

Distinguishing a nasal cold from hay fever is sometimes difficult, but the different character of the nasal discharge is revealing. Generally, if it is hay fever, the mucus is thin and colorless; if a cold is responsible, the mucus is often very thick and may be yellow or green. If fever accompanies the symptoms, an infection rather than hay fever is responsible.

The symptoms result from the presence in the air we breathe of an allergen or irritant to which we are sensitive. These particulate "aeroallergens," as they are called, are usually from 2 to 60 microns in diameter — millions of them would be needed to cover this dot (.).

Hay fever usually begins with sneezing and a runny nose. Then, as it intensifies, the eyes may run and smart, the nasal discharge becomes more copious, and the sneezing worsens to the point where it becomes incessant. Sometimes the sneezing is so persistent that it causes intense soreness and pain in the muscles of the chest and diaphragm. At this point asthmatic symptoms may appear — wheezing, difficulty in breathing, and mucus production in the airways. If not treated — or if the source is not avoided — these asthmatic symptoms can progress to the point at which they require drastic treatment.

Hay fever symptoms are at their worst when the sufferer is directly exposed to high concentrations of the allergen, whatever it is — but the problem is that, once the reaction starts, relatively low dosages of the allergen can maintain it. As a result, sleep tends to be interrupted and fitful, and there is considerable discomfort and stress associated with an attack. Hay fever is no fun. Furthermore, individuals who do not have it have no conception of the acute discomfort and the real danger it represents. One cross every hay fever sufferer has to bear is the well-meaning friend who says "bless you" and laughs every time you sneeze.

Home Treatment of Hay Fever

You can think of hay fever as fitting into any one of a number of categories according to whatever it is that causes it. The method of treatment will vary according to the triggering agent; but, in all cases, environmental control of the responsible allergens is also very important. In order to treat your hay fever, find out what you are allergic to by referring to your history and by having a physical exam and allergy skin tests (see Chapter 5). Once the causes are known, certain actions are dictated. If you are severely allergic to pollens, for instance, work to avoid those responsible for your discomfort. Find someone else to mow the lawn, keep your window closed at night, install an air purifier, even decide to take a vacation far, far away during the peak allergy season. If you are allergic to dog dander you will have to find another home for Spot and his bed; if you react to the feathers in your pillow, down sleeping bag, or comforter, you will want to revamp your sleeping arrangements. If house dust is the culprit, a vigorous program of dust removal and control is indicated.

These simple environmental measures are certainly easier, and often more successful, than drug therapy. Beyond appropriate avoidance measures, the type of treatment depends somewhat on the type of symptoms you show. (See Table 1.)

Drug Treatment of Hay Fever

For many years antihistamines have been the standard treatment for most people with mild hay fever. Most are relatively inexpensive without prescription. Some come with a decongestant, supposedly designed to help clear mucus in the nose. For most hay fever sufferers these over-the-counter (OTC) antihistamines work well enough, although they do cause some side effects, the worst being drowsiness (virtually all these medications carry the warning not to drive or operate machinery). This sedative

Type of Symptoms	Treatment(s)	Comment
Mild, seasonal	Establish and avoid cause	ASTHMA FINDER (Figure 5) may help Review Chapters 5, 6
	Use over-the-counter antihistamines as necessary and if tolerated; otherwise, use prescription nonsedating antihistamines	Be alert to possible side effects; beware of dangerous interactions with alcohol, other drugs; if asthma symptoms also present, beware of sedation
		Usually no activity limitation is necessary
Mild, chronic (year-round)	Establish and avoid cause	See above
	Invoke any necessary environmental controls	Air purifiers or conditioners can help greatly; other measures to block out or minimize allergen exposure also extremely useful
	Use prescription nonsedating antihistamines like Seldane or Hismanyl	See above
	If symptoms nagging and not helped by OTC remedies, ask physician for prescription for intranasal steroids or Nasalcrom (Nasacort, Beconase, Vancenase, Nasalide)	Must be taken at least a week before they affect symptoms. Establish and use only minimum effective dose
		Avoid activities or environments that intensify symptoms
Moderate to severe, seasonal or chronic	Establish and avoid cause	See above
	Invoke any necessary environmental controls	See above
	Use prescription medications if necessary	See above
	Get allergy shots	If allergen has been identified positively and if otherwise indicated
	Reduce exposure by limiting activities appropriately	

side effect is a mixed blessing for the sufferer who has to take antihistamines during work or study. Two new nonsedative antihistamines are now available: Seldane and Hismanyl. They relieve mild and moderate hay fever symptoms but are relatively ineffective for severe symptoms.

We have known for a long time that cortisone significantly relieves severe hay fever. Cortisone was once administered in only two ways — orally by Prednisone (a form of cortisone) for four to seven days or more prior to the start of the pollen season or by a cortisone injection once or twice during the season. Both methods have severe toxic effects. High doses or long-term use of cortisone can reduce your body's ability to fight infections, make the skin grow thin, and cause osteoporosis, or thinning of bones. It can even induce cataracts. Although these effects are unlikely if you only take corticosteroids *once,* if you take them regularly (and particularly if you begin them as a child), these side effects are quite likely to show up.

Chemists have been working to reduce cortisone toxicity for the past two decades. About 10 years ago a number of breakthroughs occurred. Chemists discovered that they could synthesize a drug like cortisone which, if sprayed in the nose, does not survive in the body for more than a few minutes and will be metabolized (destroyed) before being absorbed by the body. With these new synthetics you get the benefit of cortisone in your nose without its side effects.

We routinely recommend these intranasal steroids, or cortisone-like materials, for moderate to severe hay fever sufferers whose symptoms do not respond to, or who simply cannot tolerate, antihistamines.

> Sylvia, a law student, has had hay fever for the past eight years. Allerest, an antihistamine, helps her symptoms but makes her so sleepy she just cannot do her studies. Intranasal steroids were prescribed. Two weeks later she was back at her doctor's to celebrate. She had never felt so well during pollen season.

These medications are so effective that many physicians believe that if intranasal steroids do not work chances are good that the diagnosis of hay fever is wrong. There is one word of advice about these sprays. They are preventives and take several days to work. Don't expect your symptoms to stop immediately after a spray; relief will come along five to seven days later. Because of this delayed action, intranasal steroids must be taken regularly and in advance of need. Start them a week or two before the season commences and discontinue them as soon as the season is over.

The intranasal steroids currently on the market are Beconase, Vancenase, Nasalide, and Nasacort. Beconase and Vancenase are exactly the same product made by one company in Scotland and distributed and sold by two companies in America under their different trade names. They even carry different prices and cost about $10–$16 per canister. A canister lasts approximately three to five weeks, depending on frequency of use. Both Beconase and Vancenase contain a steroid called beclomethasone. It is usually given as one spray in each nostril two or three times a day and needs at least five days to take hold. Once it works, reduce the dose until you establish the minimum amount that will continue to control your symptoms.. After two or three weeks only one spray in each nostril daily may be enough. Nasacort, on the other hand, is effective when taken only once a day and is therefore more convenient. Unlike the other nasal sprays, Nasacort does not burn and is usually nonirritating.

Beconase, Vancenase, and Nasacort are only approved for children over 12, although many doctors ignore this limitation and frequently prescribe them for children as young as six. Nasalide, the other intranasal steroid, is a different chemical compound. It is approved for children over six and does not carry propellant. Unfortunately, it often irritates and burns the nose and for this reason many children find it intolerable. Like the other sprays it takes several days to work. The recommended starter dose is usually one spray in each nostril two or three times a day. When it gets established, determine the least amount of spray that will relieve the symptoms and discontinue when it is no longer needed.

Another development in the treatment of hay fever is a prescription nasal spray called Nasalcrom. This spray contains a solution of cromolyn sodium, the same medication used for the treatment of chronic severe asthma. It is not a steroid and has to be taken more frequently than intranasal steroids, up to four to six times daily. Nasalcrom is not as potent as intranasal steroids, but it works for most people. We find it to be a useful alternative to intranasal steroids, and, since it hardly ever burns the nose (one disadvantage of steroids), it is more readily accepted by children. A number of other intranasal steroidlike and cromolyn-like drugs for the nose will appear in the next several years.

RECURRENT EAR INFECTIONS

Many a parent knows the anguish of nights spent with a youngster with an earache. The symptoms and history are virtually the same from child to child: an infant or toddler has had a cold and a runny nose for one or two days. Suddenly, and often without warning, the child's temperature shoots up and an excruciatingly painful earache develops. Nothing the parent does pacifies the child, who becomes restless and irritable, cannot be put down, and will not sleep. The episodes last from 8 to 24 hours and generally respond to a mixture of antibiotics and decongestant therapy. Children who develop ear infections of this nature should be seen immediately by their doctor, who will look in the ear to determine if the infection is due to a virus or bacteria. If bacterial, antibiotics are given.

Children with recurrent ear infections often have a history of allergic rhinitis, or hay fever. Many also have asthma. Other children have recurrent ear infections without allergic complications or asthma.

The reason for these infections is an anatomic one. A thin tube, the Eustachian tube, which runs between the nose and the ear, is extremely small in young children. It only takes a small amount of mucus or thickening for the tube to clog up. When it does, it causes the pain and swelling of the ear drum that accompany the infection.

Regardless of the cause, the treatment of children with chronic infections is the same. Paper-thin plastic artificial tubes are placed in the ear drum to allow movement of air in the middle part of the ear. They act to help out the blocked Eustachian tube which, as the child grows older, enlarges, thus reducing the likelihood of ear infection.

Air tubes are relatively easy to install but they have some disadvantages. In very young children (less than one year old) the tubes tend to fall out. In that event, they can be placed back in the ear, but if it happens frequently the ear drum becomes too thin and flexible to support the tube. Implanting ear tubes involves a small operation, so that children must be anesthetized, which can be upsetting to both child and parent. In addition, once the tubes are implanted, some care is needed to avoid trauma. Water must be kept out, which means that swimming, taking showers, and washing hair may be a problem. Molded ear plugs are sometimes used to keep the tubes more firmly in place, but these are cumbersome and not always successful.

SINUSITIS

The sinuses are a network of hollow spaces behind the nose. They occupy most of the front of the head and drain upper airway mucus as well as act as a generalized cleanser of facial and nasal tissue. These caves are connected by narrow holes or orifices. If these orifices become blocked, as happens all too often, the caves behind them also become clogged and inflamed. The chronic inflammation that occurs in these caves, or sinuses — sinusitis — is one of the more common chronic debilitating diseases, and it is often associated with asthma and hay fever.

Individuals with sinusitis complain of a heaviness, often a bogginess, behind the nose and below the eyes. The bogginess may become so severe that a characteristic sinus headache results. If the sinus becomes infected, there may be a fever accompanied by a purulent (pus) discharge from the nose. The headache and the pain of sinusitis produce acute discomfort.

Sinusitis in asthmatics occurs much more frequently than it does in the general population, and when it does the asthma may be much more difficult to treat. This does not mean that sinusitis induces asthma; it only makes it less responsive to treatment. Moreover, the sinusitis may be chronic and silent (indolent). In other words, it may not be obvious because it has existed for so long that it goes unnoticed. Where asthma symptoms persist for no apparent reason, the possibility of sinusitis should be carefully and thoroughly considered.

The Diagnosis of Indolent Sinusitis

One of the most underutilized diagnostic procedures in the management of patients with asthma is a four-way CAT scan of the sinuses. Compared to a sinus X ray, a CAT scan provides more information, involves less radiation, and costs less. The scan reveals all the sinuses in the body, shows the size of the sinus, and indicates whether the tissue is swollen or inflamed. It may even reveal the presence of fluid within the sinus.

If your asthma becomes difficult to control, or if you have had asthma for some time seemingly without problems, and then suddenly go through a prolonged bout (often following a viral illness), and if your symptoms become stubborn, consider a CAT scan. If you have a puslike nasal discharge, a CAT scan is strongly indicated.

The Treatment of Sinusitis

There is significant disagreement among allergists and ENT (ear, nose, and throat) specialists about the best way to treat sinusitis. Allergists believe that sinusitis should be treated with a minimum of four to six weeks of antibiotic therapy. Sinus infections can be chronic and are very difficult to clear up. This is why a several-week course of antibiotics is prescribed and why your doctor will admonish you to complete the full course.

ENT physicians contend that sinus irrigation — flushing out the sinuses — should be done relatively early in patients with sinusitis. Although they may prescribe a course of antibiotics, they will go to irrigation if improvement does not occur quickly. Since approximately 50 percent of the cases do not respond to a prolonged course of antibiotics, irrigation may be required anyway. Allergists find that a full antibiotic treatment without irrigation is effective half of the time. Neither set of statistics is particularly impressive.

The Use of Nasal Sprays in Sinusitis

If we could remove any single group of drugs from your pharmacy shelves, it would be the over-the-counter sprays such as Afrin, Neosynephrine, and 4-Way designed to clear your nose and sinus passages. A common head cold may clog your sinuses and make you acutely uncomfortable. In those circumstances a brief — no more than one- or two-day — course of these nasal sprays may produce significant relief. For the patient with allergies, however, use of these drugs may become habitual. We have seen scores of asthmatics become so addicted to these sprays that they end up using them 3–10 times a day for years on end. This abuse results in a syndrome called *rhinitis medicamentosa,* which is nothing more than a swelling and constriction of the nasal passages due to the medicine itself. What occurs is that the medicine seems to work at first but, as time passes, adaptation occurs and larger and more frequent doses are required to produce an effect. A vicious cycle begins with the nose perpetually clogged unless (and sometimes even when) these nasal sprays are used. It is for that reason that we strongly discourage their use. If you suspect that you have these symptoms from overuse of nose spray, have your physician confirm the diagnosis. Once identified, the condition can be treated readily with topical steroids. (See Chapter 15, Table 12.)

The Use of Antihistamines and Decongestants in Sinusitis

For many years antihistamines and decongestants were the treatment of choice in the management of sinusitis. However, recent studies have demonstrated that these remedies do little or no good. Antihistamines, in particular, may only dry up sinus secretions and make them difficult for the patient to clear out. Decongestants may help a few individuals but are clearly not as efficacious as once believed. Antibiotics are the mainstay of and the key to successful treatment. Once the sinusitis is controlled, you and your doctor should search to find out why you developed sinusitis in the first place.

ACUTE BRONCHOPULMONARY ASPERGILLOSIS

Molds occur everywhere. If you are allergic to molds, it should be fairly obvious from your history; if not, allergy skin tests or a RAST test (discussed at the end of Chapter 5) will usually confirm it. Acute bronchopulmonary aspergillosis is found exclusively in individuals who have asthma. In this syndrome patients develop extreme allergy to the mold aspergillus, which is a genus of fungi. When skin-tested with the mold aspergillus, its victims show extremely severe reactions. Moreover, if IgE levels are determined, they are high. Finally, a special blood test for aspergillosis, called precipitating antibodies, will be positive. This condition is rare but can occur whether your asthma is recent or long-standing and regardless of your age.

> Pauline has had asthma for about 15 years. It has been well controlled with theophyllines and occasional use of Alupent. For the past two weeks she has noted a significant increase in cough and mucus production. The mucus is particularly thick and seems to be tinged with some greenish material. She feels as if she also has a fever, although the two times she took her temperature it was normal. The usual drugs she takes for asthma do not seem to work this time. Her doctor listened to her chest and thought she might have pneumonia. He ordered a chest X ray, which showed an infiltrate — some inflammation within the lung. The doctor feels fairly confident about the diagnosis of pneumonia but he remembered mention of a syndrome called acute bronchopulmonary aspergillosis. So to be on the safe side he tested her and found she did have the

condition. He treated her with a high dose of Prednisone (a steroid). Pauline took several days to respond but now feels much, much better. Six months later she is completely symptom-free. Her asthma is under control.

If Pauline's doctor had not been aware of this syndrome, two serious conditions might have developed. First, this acute hypersensitivity to the aspergillus can result in actual destruction of lung tissue. Second, it can produce abnormalities in the architecture of the air tubes, called bronchiectasis. Here the air tubes, in addition to being irritable, become tortuous, developing out-pocketings and big sacs, and so are prone to recurrent infection, making the patient's asthma much more difficult to treat.

Although it is relatively uncommon, you should know of this possibility and remind your doctor about it. If your asthma becomes more difficult and more resistant to usual treatment, or if you develop a more severe or stubborn cough, and the mucus becomes thick and tenacious and looks different from that produced during prior bouts of asthma, you may have acute bronchopulmonary aspergillosis.

CHAPTER

CHAPTER 5 Identifying the Cause of Asthma

IDENTIFYING AND CONTROLLING ASTHMA

To manage and control your asthma, you may have to take some or all of the following steps:

1. Identify the causal agents.
2. Avoid the causal agents (strategies for doing this are discussed in detail in Part 2, especially Chapter 6).
3. Control or suppress the appearance of symptoms through medication and other strategies, including desensitization (Part 3 is entirely devoted to care and control of asthma).
4. Treat symptoms with medications (Chapter 15 provides a comprehensive appraisal of the various drugs and medicines available).

What Are Asthma's Causal Agents and Which Ones Make Me Sick?

Finding the causal agent is the single most important step you can take toward controlling your asthma. Unless you establish what is making you wheeze, you will have trouble treating it and you will always be troubled by it.

There are many factors that precipitate asthma attacks. The most important ones are

- Colds or upper respiratory infections
- Allergens (dusts, pollen, molds, animal dander, etc.)
- Foods, especially food additives
- Vigorous exercise
- Emotional responses, including hyperventilation

- Certain drugs, especially aspirin and ibuprofen (Advil, Nuprin, etc.)
- Air pollutants, including tobacco smoke, smoke from wood-burning stoves, ozone, and sulfur dioxide

The surest way to pinpoint the cause of your asthma is to carefully and faithfully fill out and maintain the ASTHMA FINDER (Figure 5). This is an easy process to find out what is making you wheeze, but you must keep it up for an adequate period of time.

Begin by photocopying the ASTHMA FINDER. Fill it out every night before going to bed. It should take no more than 10 minutes.

Use the Symptoms section to assess the severity of your asthma on a given day. If you had no symptoms at all, check 0. If your symptoms were mild and did not keep you from your regular activities, check 1. If your symptoms were moderate and prevented you from carrying out *some* activities, check 2. If your symptoms were severe enough to keep you from work or school, or confined to home or bed, check 3. If your symptoms were so severe as to require hospitalization or emergency treatment, check 4.

A more objective way to assess your condition is with a peak expiratory flow (PEF) meter, a device that measures how much air you can blow out. Your physician can prescribe this tool for you, in which case your health insurance should help pay for it. See Appendix H for a list of companies that sell PEF meters, and page 133 for a picture of how to use one. Use your PEF meter twice each day, on arising and on going to bed. Grade those readings in comparison to your personal best score:

compared to best	grade	suggested response
80–100%	G (green; proceed)	No action necessary
50–80%	Y (yellow; caution)	Consider starting or increasing your medication
below 50%	R (red; danger)	Medical alert! Take a bronchodilator and notify your physician

(The percentage boundaries of G, Y, and R given here are only suggestions; work out your own parameters in consultation with your physician, based on the nature and severity of your asthma.)

In the Possible Causes section, check every item for which you had a "yes" answer that day. At the end of the week, count the checkmarks for each item and record the number in the "Total" column at the right.

To interpret the ASTHMA FINDER, relate the severity of your symptoms to the appearance of possible causes. For example, if you checked 0 in the Symptoms section all week or graded each day as G, what Possible Causes lines contain no check marks? If you did have symptoms or graded a day as Y or R, what possible causes did you notice on that day or on the day before? If you were troubled with symptoms throughout the whole week, which boxes had check marks every day? Look for patterns. Write down any suspected match of symptoms and causes.

FIGURE 5 ASTHMA FINDER

	Mon	Tue	Wed	Thu	Fri	Sat	Sun	TOTAL
How severe were your symptoms?								
No wheezing 0								
Very mild wheezing 1								
Audible wheezing 2								
Loud wheezing 3								
Severe wheezing 4								
What were your PEF AM								
readings (G,Y, or R)? PM								
When did your symptoms show?								
Morning								
Afternoon								
Evening								
During the night								
Did you have any respiratory infections?								
Cold (cough, sniffle, sore throat)								
Flu								
Sinusitis								
Other*								
Were you exposed to airborne irritants?								
Pollens								
House or other dust								
Animals/pets								
Mold								
Were you exposed to tobacco smoke?								
Were you exposed to asthma-triggering foods, beverages, or additives?								
Foods containing metabisulfite (see Appendix C)								
Foods containing tartrazine FD&C #5 (see Appendix B)								
Other possible triggers (berries, fish, mollusks, crustaceans, nuts, milk, eggs, wheat)*								
Were you exposed to asthma-triggering medications?								
Aspirin or salicylates (see Appendix D)								
Other pain or headache remedy								
Cold medications								
Nose drops								
Antibiotics								
Were you exposed to air pollution or automobile emissions?								
Were you exposed to chemicals, fumes, or odors?								
Did you exercise vigorously?								
Did you experience any asthma-triggering climatic factors?								
Brisk wind								
Cold, dry air								
Rain/snow								
Did you experience any emotional triggers?								
Stress								
Anxiety								
Conflict								

*Specify

Symptoms

Possible
Causes

for the week
of _____
to _____

_____
(name)

ASTHMA FINDER (SAMPLE)

FOR *Jennifer H.* (Name) Week of *January 14* (Month) (Date) to *21* (Date) 19*86*

Jennifer is a two-and-a-half-year-old who wheezes every day at her day care center. The day care center has three cuddly cats! Jennifer is very allergic to cat dander.

		Mon	Tue	Wed	Thu	Fri	Sat	Sun	TOTAL
How severe were your symptoms?									
No wheezing	0						✓	✓	2
Very mild wheezing	1	✓			✓				2
Audible wheezing	2		✓	✓					2
Loud wheezing	3					✓			1
Severe wheezing	4								
What were your PEF	AM	Y	R	R	Y	R	G	G	5
readings (G,Y, or R)?	PM	Y	R	Y	Y	Y	G	G	4
When did your symptoms show?									
Morning		✓	✓	✓	✓	✓			5
Afternoon		✓	✓	✓	✓	✓			5
Evening									
During the night									
Did you have any respiratory infections?									
Cold (cough, sniffle, sore throat)									
Flu									
Sinusitis									
Other*									
Were you exposed to airborne irritants?									
Pollens									
House or other dust									
Animals/pets		✓	✓	✓	✓	✓			5
Mold									
Were you exposed to tobacco smoke?									
Were you exposed to asthma-triggering foods, beverages, or additives?									
Foods containing metabisulfite (see Appendix C)									
Foods containing tartrazine FD&C #5 (see Appendix B)									
Other possible triggers (berries, fish, mollusks, crustaceans, nuts, milk, eggs, wheat)*									
Were you exposed to asthma-triggering medications?									
Aspirin or salicylates (see Appendix D)									
Other pain or headache remedy									
Cold medications									
Nose drops									
Antibiotics									
Were you exposed to air pollution or automobile emissions?									
Were you exposed to chemicals, fumes, or odors?						✓			1
Did you exercise vigorously?		✓	✓	✓	✓	✓			5
Did you experience any asthma-triggering climatic factors?									
Brisk wind									
Cold, dry air									
Rain/snow									
Did you experience any emotional triggers?									
Stress									
Anxiety									
Conflict									

*Specify

Bonnie is a twenty-nine-year-old office worker. She has had asthma all of her life and wheezes whenever in contact with virtually all the asthma triggers unless she takes her medicine.

ASTHMA FINDER (SAMPLE)

FOR _Bonnie P._   Week of ___May 6___ to _13_ _1986_
(Name)   (Month)   (Date)   (Date)

		Mon	Tue	Wed	Thu	Fri	Sat	Sun	TOTAL
How severe were your symptoms?									
No wheezing	0	✓			✓	✓			3
Very mild wheezing	1						✓	✓	2
Audible wheezing	2			✓					1
Loud wheezing	3				✓				1
Severe wheezing	4								
What were your PEF	AM	G	Y	R	G	G	Y	Y	3
readings (G,Y, or R)?	PM	G	G	Y	G	Y	Y	Y	5
When did your symptoms show?									
Morning				✓			✓	✓	3
Afternoon				✓					1
Evening			✓	✓					2
During the night			✓	✓					2
Did you have any respiratory infections?									
Cold (cough, sniffle, sore throat)									
Flu									
Sinusitis									
Other*									
Were you exposed to airborne irritants?									
Pollens		✓	✓	✓	✓	✓	✓	✓	7
House or other dust									
Animals/pets									
Mold									
Were you exposed to tobacco smoke?		✓	✓	✓	✓	✓	✓	✓	7
Were you exposed to asthma-triggering foods, beverages, or additives?									
Foods containing metabisulfite (see Appendix C)				✓					1
Foods containing tartrazine FD&C #5 (see Appendix B)									
Other possible triggers (berries, fish, mollusks, crustaceans, nuts, milk, eggs, wheat)*									
Were you exposed to asthma-triggering medications?									
Aspirin or salicylates (see Appendix D)									
Other pain or headache remedy									
Cold medications									
Nose drops									
Antibiotics									
Were you exposed to air pollution or automobile emissions?									
Were you exposed to chemicals, fumes, or odors?									
Did you exercise vigorously?			✓	✓			✓	✓	4
Did you experience any asthma-triggering climatic factors?									
Brisk wind									
Cold, dry air									
Rain/snow									
Did you experience any emotional triggers?									
Stress									
Anxiety									
Conflict: _Argument with boyfriend_							✓	✓	2

*Specify

ASTHMA FINDER (SAMPLE)

FOR ___Tod___ Week of ___February 3___ to ___10___ 19 86
(Name) (Month) (Date) (Date)

Tod is a fourth-grade student. He wheezes whenever he has a cold. His dad is a chain smoker.

	Mon	Tue	Wed	Thu	Fri	Sat	Sun	TOTAL
How severe were your symptoms?								
No wheezing 0	✓							1
Very mild wheezing 1		✓					✓	2
Audible wheezing 2						✓		1
Loud wheezing 3			✓					1
Severe wheezing 4				✓	✓			2
What were your PEF AM	G	Y	R	R	R	Y	Y	6
readings (G,Y, or R)? PM	Y	R	R	R	Y	Y	Y	7
When did your symptoms show?								
Morning				✓	✓	✓		3
Afternoon				✓	✓	✓		3
Evening			✓	✓	✓	✓		4
During the night		✓	✓	✓	✓	✓	✓	6
Did you have any respiratory infections?								
Cold (cough, sniffle, sore throat)	✓	✓	✓	✓				4
Flu								
Sinusitis								
Other*								
Were you exposed to airborne irritants?								
Pollens								
House or other dust								
Animals/pets								
Mold								
Were you exposed to tobacco smoke?	✓	✓	✓	✓	✓	✓	✓	7
Were you exposed to asthma-triggering foods, beverages, or additives?								
Foods containing metabisulfite (see Appendix C)								
Foods containing tartrazine FD&C #5 (see Appendix B)								
Other possible triggers (berries, fish, mollusks, crustaceans, nuts, milk, eggs, wheat)*								
Were you exposed to asthma-triggering medications?								
Aspirin or salicylates (see Appendix D)								
Other pain or headache remedy								
Cold medications	✓	✓		✓				3
Nose drops								
Antibiotics								
Were you exposed to air pollution or automobile emissions?								
Were you exposed to chemicals, fumes, or odors?								
Did you exercise vigorously?	✓							1
Did you experience any asthma-triggering climatic factors?								
Brisk wind								
Cold, dry air		✓	✓					2
Rain/snow	✓							1
Did you experience any emotional triggers?								
Stress								
Anxiety								
Conflict								

*Specify

47

You may have to keep the ASTHMA FINDER for a number of weeks (photocopy the form), but stay with it. It's your best tool for identifying what is making you sick.

The following seven tips may help you in your search for the causal agent or agents that are responsible for your asthma.

1. *Colds or upper respiratory infections* are by far the most common forerunners of asthmatic attacks in children. The cold symptoms — sneezing, sniffling, coughing, stuffy nose, sore throat, possibly a slight fever — usually appear before asthma takes hold. Then the congestion will get worse, the chest will feel constricted, and shortness of breath, deeper coughing, and wheezing will show up. These asthmatic symptoms may persist well after the main infection is gone.

Pat's asthma started in childhood and has never disappeared. Although she often goes several months between episodes, the way her wheezing begins is exactly the same now at age 43 as it was at age 6. Whenever she develops a cold, stuffy nose, or sore throat, with or without a fever, in a few hours to a couple of days she begins to feel her chest tightening up. The sequence is so invariant and predictable that she has learned to take her asthma medications at the first sign of a cold. This often significantly reduces, if not entirely prevents, the wheezing that accompanies a cold. She also knows that she has to continue to take her medications for two to three weeks following a cold. During the fall and winter seasons, when colds or flu are going around, Pat takes the medication even though she is not ill — a simple precaution, but it works. And at the first sign of spring she shelves her medication.

2. *Up to half of all asthmatics show allergies* to pollens, house dust, animals, or molds, but these allergies do not necessarily produce asthmatic reactions. They will, however, if you have a high level of IgE or if you have twitchy airways.

Gabe remembers his first summer at camp. That was the year his mother kept reminding the counselor that Gabe had allergies and needed to take his medication every day without fail. When asked what Gabe was allergic to, his mother replied, "All living things."

Gabe had a fine time that summer; he also learned that he was not allergic "to all living things." Grass pollens, he discovered, were responsible for his symptoms. Whenever he was exposed to them and not shielded by his medication, the IgE response led to wheezing and shortness of breath. When away from pollen, or appropriately medicated, Gabe had no problems at all.

If your asthma is due to this class of allergens, tracking down the one or ones responsible will be greatly helped if you keep in mind that the symptoms are likely to come around at about the same time each year, they are prone to aggravation by conditions that put particulate material in the air you breathe (brisk winds; sweeping the garage; riding with the car windows open), and they are apt to turn up after a visit to the same physical location. If you always get wheezy when you drop in on Aunt Grace and her houseful of cats, the felines probably have something to do with your symptoms.

3. *Foods* draw much unwarranted suspicion as causes of asthma. The popular idea that your asthma can be provoked by some mysterious, insidious allergy to foods is largely unfounded — foods seldom cause asthma. *Food additives* can and do, though, particularly tartrazine, which is found in food dye color #5 (FDC#5), a yellow dye used in potato chips, tacos, and other yellow candy and processed foods. Foods containing tartrazine are listed in Appendix B.

Another additive, metabisulfite, a food preservative, is increasingly evident as an asthma provoker. Foods containing metabisulfite are listed in Appendix C.

> Alan has had asthma all of his life. He controls it by taking theophylline daily and occasionally using an aerosol. However, on several recent occasions he developed an intense cough, sometimes cutting short special evenings out with his wife. Alan began to keep a record listing everything he had eaten leading up to the appearance of this cough. He and his wife had visited several restaurants, and dined on dishes from many different food groups. Then Alan realized that the cough usually appeared after he drank wine. He took his notes to his physician. After reviewing the history, the doctor concluded that Alan was reacting to metabisulfite, a preserving agent in widespread use which is added to many wines. Since then, Alan has avoided wine, and no longer has the acute episodes of asthma associated with metabisulfite. He and his wife have enjoyed many more relaxed evenings together.

If you think that food allergy is triggering your asthma, Chapter 7 spells out the steps to take to track down the culprit.

4. *Vigorous exercise* is frequently implicated in bronchospasm. Interestingly, the form of exercise has much to do with it. Swimming is relatively harmless and unlikely to provoke airway collapse in asthmatics, while running or jogging often will. Whether or not exercise will cause you to wheeze depends on the temperature and humidity of the air you breathe — the moister and the warmer the air, the less the likelihood that you will have a bronchospasm. Exercise and asthma are discussed in detail in Chapter 9.

5. *Emotional responses* — anger and fear in particular — have long been blamed for causing asthma. Whereas emotional states like anger and resentment do not *induce* asthma, they often cause rapid, shallow breathing, or hyperventilation. This hyperventilation in individuals with twitchy airways ends in bronchospasm and wheezing. There are probably other ways in which emotional reactions following conflict, stress, or danger can induce bronchospasm, but the reasons for these and the ways in which they act are still unknown.

6. *Many drugs*, particularly those classified as nonsteroidal anti-inflammatory drugs (aspirin, ibuprofen, Advil, Nuprin, Motrin, and their relatives), can provoke violent asthmatic reactions. If you have asthma, steer clear of aspirin and all other nonsteroidal drugs. The package label or your pharmacist will tell you whether or not your pain relief medicine fits in this category.

Grant has suffered from asthma on and off all of his life. He has never exactly figured out the cause of his asthma, because most of the time it is not so bad. However, he noticed that he would wheeze with a cold, especially one where a fever was present. Grant and his doctor concluded that the asthma symptoms were associated with more severe infections. However, Grant became suspicious after reading news stories about the possible role of aspirin in inducing Reye's syndrome in children. Grant, an adult, could not get Reye's syndrome, but he still wondered about aspirin because he routinely took it for bad colds.

When Grant inquired further, his doctor affirmed that aspirin can make asthma worse in some people. With his suspicions aroused, the doctor had Grant take a small amount of aspirin after doing some pulmonary function tests. He waited a short time, and then repeated the tests. On retrial, Grant's pulmonary function tests' performance decreased slightly, although Grant felt the same and could not believe that he was having some collapse of his airways. However, during a viral cold, airways tend to collapse anyway, and the cumulative effect of the aspirin and the infection was enough to tip Grant over the edge until he became symptomatic. Grant now uses acetaminophen when he has a cold and fever.

7. There have been a number of notorious incidents of serious *air pollution* in industrial areas causing epidemic respiratory illness and death. The dense smog in London in December 1952 was one such event. During this episode air samples showed a tenfold increase in concentration of sulfur dioxide and particulate matter. Studies done in London as well as subsequent ones in the Meuse Valley in France and in Donora, Pennsylvania, showed that 88 percent of asthmatic people develop respiratory symptoms during these air inversions. Apparently sulfur dioxide, ozone, and the particulate pollutants resulting from the combustion of fossil fuels cause twitchy airways to get worse. In fact, virtually anyone, asthmatic or not, will develop bronchospasm from sulfur dioxide. However, because of the hypersensitivity of their airways, asthmatics react severely. They become quite sick at concentrations of sulfur dioxide too low to affect people without asthma.

In addition to atmospheric pollutants, tobacco smoke — first- or second-hand — is an important triggering agent for asthma and should be studiously avoided.

ALLERGY TESTS

If you use the ASTHMA FINDER carefully and conscientiously, you should be able to pick out what is causing your wheezing. In the event that it fails to come up with the cause, you may want — or your doctor may recommend — a series of allergy tests in the doctor's office to identify the agent responsible for your illness.

Before submitting to a course of tests to try to pin down the source of your asthma,

than prick tests. Twenty minutes after injection the site is reexamined and measured for wheal and flare.

The grading systems used to evaluate the wheal and flare response to either prick or intradermal tests are likely to vary from one physician to another. In order to standardize observations, however, in addition to the suspected allergens, two comparison tests are made. A substance known to produce a strong positive reaction (usually histamine) is administered; and one that does not cause a wheal and flare response (usually saline solution) is also given. These two tests help define the limits of your reactions and make it certain that your tests can be interpreted accurately.

Which skin tests are given should be determined in part by where you live. Skin tests can be divided into several categories. First, and probably the most common, are those using *pollens*. They consist of extracts of trees, weeds, and grasses. Obviously you should be skin tested with local pollens. Generally allergists screen with the full panel of tests, even if your history suggests only grass sensitivity, in order to be complete and to find out how atopic you are. Second, there are the *mold antigens*; molds are found almost everywhere, and many asthmatics are allergic to them. Third are the *environmental agents* which include things found in the home — especially house dust and animal danders. Finally, there are extracts available for skin testing that claim to detect *sensitivity to certain foods. These last tests should rarely be used; they are very crude and quite unlikely to yield clinically important information.* If foods are suspected, then the physician should carry out a special challenge test, as described in Chapter 7.

Interpreting Skin Tests

The interpretation of skin tests results is a complex and tricky affair. For one thing, skin tests do not always coincide with clinical symptoms, although they can be informative when appropriate allergens have been selected for testing and when the results are carefully tied to your history. However, there are some special circumstances and problems that may make interpretation extremely difficult. Individuals who have dermatographism — a skin so sensitive that it develops erythema (redness) when touched or stroked — will react positively to *everything*, including the negative control (the saline). For them, skin tests are useless. In addition, for individuals with skin diseases such as eczema and psoriasis, skin tests cannot or perhaps should not be done. (See Table 2.) Skin tests are expensive. Costs vary widely; the bill for allergy skin tests can run upwards of $100–$300. Finally, there are children who cannot tolerate skin tests. Some adults are frightened by the process and simply balk at it — even though it is painless, nondisfiguring, and, when properly supervised, carries little or no risk.

TABLE 2   When to Avoid Skin Tests

Condition	Reason
Infancy (age 2 years or less)	Not likely to be positive
Where eczema or psoriasis is present	May irritate the skin severely
Dermatographism (a condition in which the skin reddens and swells following pressure)	Tests cannot be interpreted
Use of antihistamines	Antihistamines block the skin test

Eighteen-year-old Eric has had hay fever for the past 12 years. He takes over-the-counter antihistamines and, except for feeling sleepy, is generally comfortable and in control of his seasonal symptoms. However, during a really bad allergy year, and on a windy day, he notices that he wheezes a bit. He decided to see his doctor about this. His doctor thought Eric would be a good candidate for allergy shots. He knew from his history that Eric most likely had mild extrinsic asthma due to pollen.

Eric had a battery of skin tests containing antigens from trees, grass, weeds, molds, dusts, and animal danders. He reacted to eight of the tests, all grass antigens. The results confirmed why Eric's wheezing was always at its worst during the grass pollen season — and what grasses were to blame. The doctor considered advising Eric to have allergy shots to desensitize him to the pollen. They finally agreed that, since Eric's discomfort lasted only about six weeks, it was foolish to have him undergo an expensive series of allergy shots. Eric's problem was self-limiting and could be readily handled by medication.

Bronchial Challenge Testing for Asthma

If you believe you have allergy-induced asthma, which skin testing failed to diagnose, you may be one of the very small number of individuals for whom a technique known as bronchial challenge is appropriate. It may also be utilized if you have a special and peculiar asthma history that suggests sensitivity to a chemical found only in your workplace. If you show no symptoms on vacations or days off from work, if you feel well when you wake up in the morning, for instance, and feel well at work, but several hours after returning home begin to wheeze, an occupational irritant may be affecting you.

In such instances — especially where disability and workman's compensation is an issue or when workers have to consider retraining and reemployment — bronchial challenge tests can pick out the offending allergen. They are administered when you are free of symptoms and not taking medication. You are first asked to inhale a saline mist solution so that a baseline measurement of pulmonary function can be obtained. (Your pulmonary function is measured as you exhale into a flow meter, which records the amount and velocity of air you expel from your lungs.) The test solution is then administered when you inhale a nebulized spray — a fine, foglike mist. Graded doses of the antigen are administered in this way with pulmonary function tests repeated after each dose. The pulmonary function test establishes if a reduction in air flow correlates with the inhalation of a given antigen. This test is expensive and should only be performed by experienced physicians either in a clinic with immediate access to emergency room equipment or, preferably, by overnight admission to the hospital. The reason for this is that in rare instances severe reactions requiring emergency treatment can show up. Standardized procedures beginning with an extremely dilute solution of antigen have been worked out, however, and such serious reactions almost never occur.

Laboratory Tests for Allergies

There are two alternatives to skin testing: radioallergoabsorbent tests (RAST) and similar tests done by fluorescence (FAST). These directly measure specific IgE antibodies in the blood. Reactions to skin tests vary in intensity according to individual responsiveness, type of skin, current use of other medications, or hormonal state. RAST and FAST tests have little such individual variation. These tests, which are more expensive than skin tests, are done by drawing blood samples and sending them to a central laboratory for analysis.

The ease, simplicity, and specificity of skin testing makes it the procedure of choice, despite its extra discomfort when compared to a single blood sample needed for RAST or FAST. Moreover, results of skin testing are known within minutes; you may have to wait weeks to get the results of the RAST and FAST. Finally, the RAST and FAST tests are still being researched and refined; it is hoped that further improvements will produce a more efficient way of detecting the presence of IgE antibodies. Nonetheless, you should know that RAST and FAST do exist and may be recommended for you.

Other Blood Tests

There are other blood tests being developed or advocated for the diagnosis of allergies. One such test is the *basophil degranulation test*. It is unlikely that your doctor will order this test, since it is most commonly employed at research centers or laboratories. In this test, blood samples are taken and the white cells isolated. The suspected allergen is added directly to these white cells, and they are observed to see if they undergo degranulation and release histamine.

Another more commonly ordered test is called *total serum IgE*. This is a test that has some limited value but tends to be overused, simply because there are many people with severe allergies who have normal levels of IgE, just as there are many people who do not show any allergies at all who have high levels of IgE. The reason for this discrepancy is simply that IgE levels fluctuate for a variety of reasons other than allergies. Individuals with parasitic infestations, such as worms, may show extraordinarily high levels of IgE. Physicians may order total serum IgE to help in their baseline evaluations or to diagnose a unique complication of asthma called allergic bronchopulmonary aspergillosis, a rare but dangerous condition discussed earlier in Chapter 4.

Unhappily, certain other blood "tests" have enjoyed some vogue. Prominent among these are the collection of so-called cytotoxic tests, also known as "cytotoxicity," "leukocyte antigen sensitivity," "leukocytotoxicity," "Bryan's," or simply "food sensitivity" testing. These tests have been found to be useless — even dangerous — in diagnosis and treatment. They do not identify the hidden causes of allergic symptoms and should not be employed. There is also a long list of unproven medical tests that may be used by unscrupulous practitioners.

AVOIDING ASTHMA'S COMMON AND UNCOMMON CAUSES AND COMPLICATIONS

Avoiding the Cause of Your Asthma

The best and most effective rule for asthmatics is to avoid whatever is causing symptoms. In practice this is harder to do than it sounds because some agents (like colds and air pollution) are impossible to stay away from; others, especially additives to food, are too ubiquitous to avoid.

GENERAL STRATEGIES

The tactics you follow depend on the causal agent. For instance, if your asthma results from colds or respiratory infections, doing whatever you can to stay away from individuals who can infect you is obviously appropriate. If this means leaving a particular place — a classroom, or the workplace, for example — or if it requires that you take preventive strategies like wearing a mask, then do it. The explanation or apology is easier than another bout of the wheezes.

When drugs, foods, or food additives or preservatives are responsible for your asthma, make a point of knowing exactly what you are ingesting. Read the labels on packages, ask to know exactly what is in restaurant food, and make specific inquiries about the presence of those things that trigger your symptoms. This program of vigilance should be followed unfailingly. Resist social pressure that forces you into activities that have predictably bad results. If you know that vigorous exercise on a cold day will leave you gasping for breath, put your own needs and condition first. If somebody offers you a potato chip and you crave it desperately, go ahead and eat it — but only after you have determined that it is free of tartrazine (if tartrazine is your nemesis). If the package does not list the ingredients, refuse it.

Appendix H lists sources of a wide range of products expressly designed and manufactured for the asthmatic. It will be especially useful to you if your asthma is extrinsic in form or severe enough to require special equipment for dispensing medication.

The price of avoiding or minimizing exposure to asthma-producing agents is eternal and unfailing watchfulness, along with a measure of self-denial and discomfort. The payoff is that you will ultimately find your disease less debilitating and intrusive.

AIRBORNE ALLERGENS

Four major airborne allergens may provoke asthma — pollens, dust, animal danders, and molds.

One important avoidance tactic is to remove the offending substance from the air you breathe by means of an air filtering or purifying device. At one time wearing surgical masks or inserting bulky, uncomfortable, disfiguring sterling silver screening devices in the nostrils was routinely recommended. Today more efficient procedures are available.

Air purifiers in the home or workplace can be effective against pollens and dust, and they provide an excellent first line of defense against other airborne allergens as well. An effective air filtration system and vigorous environmental precautions are preferable to the risk, inconvenience, expense, and (all too often) ineffectiveness of an immunological program or heavy dosages of medication and drugs.

> Merle is an active, lively man of 70. But up until 20 years ago his life-style was severely hampered by asthma. Each spring he spent a lot of time at the hospital getting emergency treatment for severe attacks caused by pollen. His problem was that he was allergic to many of the wild grasses that flourished in the area where he lived. Allergy shots did not help. In retrospect, he believes it was because there were so many pollens that he reacted to. Medications did not keep him out of the emergency room when conditions were especially bad.
>
> Merle and his wife built a new home in 1973, and his physician suggested he have an air purifier installed. This wasn't too expensive because the house was going to have central air conditioning anyway. The results, then and ever since, were nothing short of sensational. While Merle still has some seasonal problems, he is able to control them with aerosols. The air filtration system paid for itself in its first year alone, just in saved emergency room costs.

There are a large number and variety of filtration or air purification systems available to remove particulate material — dust and pollens in particular — from the air. These systems may use one or a combination of filtering devices and may range in size from small units (designed for use in a confined space such as a small office) to centralized systems intended to take care of an entire house. Table 3 summarizes the various filtration systems used, their approximate cost, and other data. If, after careful study and consultation with your physician, you determine that you need such a system, keep in mind the following points:

1. Medical supply firms stock an inventory of these devices. Some permit customers to try out units prior to rental or purchase. Ask if this is possible. If not, rent for a period. (Remember that rental or purchase costs are a tax-deductible medical expense). *Try before buying!*

2. To be effective, a purifier should recirculate the air *at least* four times an hour. Thus, a unit to be placed in a 12-by-15-foot room (with an 8-foot ceiling) would have to have a capacity of not less than 100 cubic feet per minute.

3. Tightly fitting window filters that help screen out larger particles are a useful adjunct to air conditioning or purifying devices.

4. Pay close attention to the specifications of equipment you rent or purchase. There are unscrupulous manufacturers in the medical supply field who will misrepresent their merchandise.

5. Units may be purchased from large general merchandising firms like Sears and J. C. Penney. If you decide to purchase, be sure to match the

TABLE 3   Type, Operation, Costs, and Maintenance of Air Purifying Devices

Filter Type	Operating Principle	Purchase Price	Monthly Rental	Filter Costs	Maintenance	Comment
Electrostatic or electronic	Precipitates particles on electrostatically charged filter	$300 and up	$40 and up	N/A	Wash filter regularly	Some noise; produces ozone which is an irritant
HEPA (High Efficiency Particulate Arresting)	Traps particles in an extremely fine screen	$400 and up	$45 and up	$40 – $80	Replace filter every 18 months	Some noise
Fiber	Traps particles in a fine screen	$100 and up	$15 and up	$5 – $20	Replace filter monthly	Some noise; not as efficient as HEPA; some models of little or no use
Ionizing	Gives particles a negative charge which causes them to attach to positively charged surfaces	Up to $100	Up to $15	N/A	Clear surfaces attracting negatively charged particles	Quiet; units small, more than one may be needed for larger spaces

NOTE: Other types may combine various types of filters or traps; some may also incorporate activated charcoal pads which remove tobacco smoke.

specifications of the unit you are buying to those of the one you have already tried out and found useful.

6. There is an excellent summary of the pros and cons of air purifying devices in *Consumer Reports* for February, 1989. Ask for it at your local library.

Additional Tips on Avoiding Exposure to Airborne Irritants

1. Use furniture and surfaces that do not attract or hold particles. Avoid overstuffed furniture or irritant-holding fabrics like plush. Use hypoallergenic covers over the mattress of the bed, if necessary (Appendix H names suppliers). Steer clear of feather or down pillows or coverings. Books are dust or mold catchers and should be kept clean and dry.

2. Where mold is the culprit, dryness is especially important in the living/sleeping area. Use a dehumidifier. Eliminate patches of damp, especially in basement or closet areas. (An electric light of small wattage left burning in closets will often control mold or mildew). Silica gel or exposed crystals of dichlorobenzene will rid the house of fungi; they should be used with caution, and the area in which they are used should be aired completely before being inhabited again.

3. Cleanliness is important, especially in regard to animal dander. For an asthmatic, the best rule to follow is to keep only the kinds of pets that do not produce dander — goldfish, for example. (And, even then, be sure the fish tank is not putting mold into the air!) Birds, dogs, cats, rodents, and horses can and do provoke severe reactions in susceptible individuals. If you must own a pet, keep it outside.

> Dr. Mercer was invited to become the Dean at West Coast College. He had no sooner arrived at his new location in a small California city when he became seriously ill with a violent reaction to horse dander. The whole area was "horse country," and there was no place he could find to live that was free of the material in the air. His sensitivity was so great that he was forced to decline the offer and return to his former position, which had neither the salary nor the prestige of the new post, but at least did not have him fighting for breath all of the time.

Avoiding House Dust

Avoiding house dust can be extremely difficult. If you are allergic to house dust or if it makes your asthma worse, you will find the following suggestions helpful:

In General

- Avoid furniture, appliances, and decor likely to harbor dust — specifically, upholstered or ornately carved furniture, bed canopies, rugs, hanging plants (and their containers), fabric wall hangings or tapestries, knick-knack shelves, fabric lamp shades, books, stuffed animals, flocked wallpaper.

- Be alert to dust gathering on electrical or electronic equipment — light fixtures, radios, TVs, hi-fi — and on radiators and in heating vents.
- Use hard-finished nonretentive surfaces — bare wood, metal, plastic, synthetics, cotton, fiberglass.
- Rather than vacuum, dust daily with a damp mop or sponge. Use only canister or tank-type vacuums, or a central vacuum cleaning system with the collection tank in the garage. An asthmatic should not vacuum or should wear a mask while doing so.

In the Bedroom

- Remove all carpeting, wall hangings or decorations, books, and other dust collectors; store clothing in cleaned, closed closet.
- Replace curtains, drapes, and Venetian blinds with roll-down window shades; replace upholstered furniture with plain wood or plastic pieces.
- Use air purification systems, such as HEPA (see Table 3).
- Use synthetic or tightly encased pillows.
- Avoid down or feather comforters or pillows and wool blankets.
- Wash blankets frequently (every 2 – 4 weeks); damp or oil-mop floors daily; dust drawers, closets, window sills, shelves, and other surfaces daily with a damp cloth or sponge.
- Air condition if possible; keep relative humidity low (50 percent or less) to control dust mites.
- Avoid stuffed animals as much as possible. Even an innocent teddy bear can be a problem.

Kathy is four years old and has had asthma almost since birth. Kathy's room is about as dust-free as you could ever make it. There are no shelves, rugs, or curtains, and the mattress has a hypoallergenic cover. However, Kathy insists on taking her stuffed teddy bear to bed with her every night. Her mother has long suspected the bear, who looks like an overgrown shag rug, of being the dust spreader. Kathy's mom blames the bear for the nighttime wheezes. She discussed the problem with her pediatrician, who suggested that Kathy be "introduced" to a new bear, one that was washable or could be cleaned with a damp cloth. Kathy spurned the new teddy at first, but slowly her mother, by playing house with Kathy and her bears, arranged a permanent vacation for Kathy's dear old bear.

AVOIDING FOOD AND FOOD ADDITIVES

The simplest means of avoiding a particular food — or more likely, food additive or contaminant — that causes your asthma is self-evident: DON'T EAT IT. So long as you exercise a certain amount of vigilance and caution, you should be able to maintain a ban on the offending item or items. Find out in advance exactly what you are going to eat by reading labels thoroughly and carefully. Ask questions. Don't be tempted and don't relax your guard! However, there are some complicating factors you may encounter:

- The offending food or substance may occur in unexpected places. Milk, responsible for some asthmatic symptoms in susceptible individuals, turns up in everything from bologna to zabaglione; tartrazine (yellow food dye #5) is apparently put into everything processed or prepared; metabisulfite, a preservative, finds its way into alcoholic beverages and some foods susceptible to spoilage. See Appendixes B, C, and D for advice on spotting such additives.
- The offender may come from a big family. Cross-sensitivity happens frequently in food intolerances so that, if peanut butter makes you wheeze, all of the other members of the legume family such as beans and peas may do this too. Appendix E lists the members of the groups of foods that cross-react.
- In addition to the food itself or to additives intended to enhance appearance or reduce spoilage, food contaminants may also trigger asthmatic reactions. Insecticides and herbicides often turn up in fresh or processed fruits and vegetables; steroids and antibiotics are found in almost all commercially produced meats and fowl; fish taken from polluted or contaminated sources may have a high enough concentration of heavy metals or insecticide residues to cause an asthmatic reaction.

Identifying these asthma-provokers may be a bit tricky, but here again your best and surest bet is to keep a careful, systematic, thoughtful record of what you consume and to relate that to your symptoms. The ASTHMA FINDER (Figure 5) in Chapter 5 will help you. See also Chapter 7 for a more detailed discussion of diet and asthma.

REDUCING COLDS AND INFECTIONS

Avoiding exposure to colds and respiratory infections is fairly difficult. To the parents of asthmatic children, it seems as if kids are always coming down with one more cold that slips into still another asthma attack. Between the ages of two and four, children have an average of 10 to 15 colds a year. It is impossible to prevent yourself from getting a cold. In fact, repeated colds may in the long run be good for you by helping you to develop resistance to them. You may, however, be able to reduce the number and severity of your colds, as well as make your body more able to fight them, by following these precautions:

- Maintain generally good health habits: plenty of sleep, adequate diet, and so on.
- Stay in good physical shape. Follow a regular program of exercise. (See Chapter 9 for exercise appropriate for the asthmatic.)

- Avoid contact with someone who is coughing or sneezing.
- Do not get overheated.
- Drink lots of fluids.
- Avoid drafts.
- Do your breathing exercises faithfully. (Breathing exercises are described in Chapter 14.)
- Ask your doctor whether you are a candidate for a flu shot or a pneumovax vaccination.
- Wash your hands frequently during the day and keep them out of your mouth and eyes.
- Children should be helped to follow these guidelines. In addition, teach them not to share utensils or glasses, to avoid public drinking fountains, and to cover their mouths when they cough or sneeze.

If you or your child's infection is from a virus (and this is most often the case) *stay away from antibiotics.* They will not help the cold and can cause a reaction besides.

Using Home Vaporizers Effectively

Pediatricians have been recommending the use of vaporizers at home to treat colds and croupy coughs for more than 50 years. Vaporizers come in a variety of forms but all operate on the same principle. A reservoir is filled with water, air is blown into the water to generate a vapor mist, and the vaporizer is turned toward the mouth and nose so that the air inhaled contains a high concentration of water vapor. In some units the water is heated and puts out warm vapor.

Vaporizers are popular because they definitely help a croupy cough. They are inexpensive, generally less than $25, and with care will last for years. However, there are two major problems you should be aware of:

1. The cough of patients with asthma is a very different cough from the one seen in a child who has croup. An asthma cough reflects collapse of airways or bronchospasm and is not likely to be helped significantly by vapor alone.
2. The continued addition of water to vaporizers almost always forms a thick coating of mold and bacteria in the reservoir, especially in the tubes and equipment that vaporize the air. The vapor put out by such a machine is a fine mist of mold and germs. Obviously this is the last thing you want to breathe, because it may trigger an allergy and make your asthma worse.

Alice has had asthma associated with colds since she was 18 months of age. Her mother took her to a succession of doctors over the years. All prescribed medication to be started at the time her cold began and continued for about a week or two thereafter. Alice is now primarily troubled by recurrent sinusitis. Following every cold she is virtually certain to develop a sinus infection. None of her doctors understood why each and every cold ended with sinusitis.

She was referred to a nearby medical school where the allergist asked her mother if they used a vaporizer. They did. The allergist had the vaporizer brought to the clinic and examined. Although the mother insisted that she cleaned the vaporizer once a week with vinegar, she was astounded to see the ugly residue in the metal tubes above the reservoir.

Acting on the doctor's advice, Alice's mother discarded the vaporizer. Now, although Alice continues to have colds and occasional bouts of sinusitis, they are much less frequent than before. Alice continues to wheeze after exposure to damp environments, and she can never go into the basement of her home without becoming acutely uncomfortable. A repeat visit to her allergist led to allergy skin tests, which found that she was extraordinarily sensitive to molds.

We recommend judicious use of a vaporizer for very small children (below the age of six) who have croupy coughs. Do not continue its use if it does not seem to work. Moreover, remember to clean all parts of it every day.

We are often asked if a warm vapor is better than a cold one. There is no clinical difference in terms of which is better, but there are numerous instances of serious burns resulting from the hot mist type. Accordingly, we recommend vaporizers that do not heat the water.

AVOIDING EXERCISE-INDUCED ASTHMA ATTACKS

If vigorous exercise such as jogging or bicycling pushes you into an asthmatic attack, you have three choices: exercise anyway and suffer the consequences, take up another activity that does not leave you sick when you finish it, or take medication beforehand.

Matthew has had asthma all of his 15 years. He is particularly troubled by wheezing during physical exercise in school and is unable to keep up with the other teens on account of it. His doctor says that he has exercise-induced asthma and has recommended that he take theophylline, which is almost invariably helpful. (See Chapter 15.) Unfortunately, Matthew is one of the few individuals who cannot tolerate theophylline. It gives him nausea, and he would much rather avoid exercise than take the medication. Matthew's parents consulted another physician, who recommended that he use a Ventolin inhaler prior to exercise. (Ventolin and other beta agonists are also discussed in Chapter 15.) Although school rules forbid students to carry hand-held nebulizers in their pockets, they do make it available in the school nurse's office, so Matthew goes there immediately before gym class. Since he started doing this he has improved greatly in stamina and, to his immense satisfaction, his athletic skills have picked up too.

As we noted in Chapter 5, it helps to avoid situations where exercise is done under cold, dry conditions or requires sustained, breath-taking effort. We cannot emphasize too strongly the value of every asthmatic learning to swim and to swim often. Swimming is an excellent form of exercise for asthmatics; several recent Olympic medalists in swimming were asthmatics. (Chapter 9 covers asthma and exercise fully.)

COPING WITH EMOTIONAL STRESS

Because of the chronic nature of their disease, asthmatics are particularly susceptible to emotional stress. The severity of the symptoms and the way in which they make the ordinary act of breathing shallow and labored are enough to trigger hyperventilation out of fear. Added to that are a myriad of other emotional upsets, which grow out of the complex and often troubled relationships that plague families of asthmatics. Asthmatics or their parents unnecessarily experience frustration, panic, and self-blame over the attacks; asthmatics, particularly children, are often frightened by attacks and spend a lot of time wondering if, this time, they are going to die. They need solicitous and understanding care and reassurance to counter this private dread. Sometimes parents and nonasthmatic siblings openly resent the attention, care, and expense that the asthmatic requires. Explaining the nature of the disease and the reasons for the preferential treatment goes a long way toward counteracting this source of tension.

At the same time, parents may increase a child's insecurity and anxiety by being oversolicitous and overprotective. As a result, they discourage their offspring from participating in and enjoying ordinary activities and thus from developing normally. In doing this they forge an undesirably close dependency, which may be difficult to break in later life, and may teach the child to use his/her condition to have his/her own way in the family or elsewhere. Maintaining a proper balance between effective care of asthmatic symptoms on the one hand and the most nearly normal development of the child on the other is extraordinarily difficult and requires patience, understanding, and the willingness to take some risks.

Here are a few tips that will help you or your child to avoid some of the major difficulties growing out of emotional responses.

- Keep lines of communication open. Discuss problems frankly and directly as they come up. Do not let them fester.
- Do not think of yourself as an invalid. With some thought and care you can do just about anything anyone else can.
- Do not treat your asthmatic children as invalids. If you do, they may start believing you.
- If there is stress or tension on the job, at home, or in school, try to locate and get rid of the reasons. (This does not mean that you need to quit, for instance. Try to talk to your boss about your difficulty and what you need to manage it.)
- Control stress or tension by slowing yourself down. Breathing exercises, meditation, or other tension-reducing activities may work for you.
- Get outside help if you find yourself consistently unhappy, depressed, or anxious. Friends, ministers, priests, social workers, psychologists, counselors, and doctors are all appropriate people to talk with.

- If your child or lover or friend is the asthmatic, strive to establish a harmonious atmosphere with easy give and take. Work to avoid stress, conflict, and anger.
- Under *no* circumstances should you, the asthmatic, take sedatives or tranquilizers to reduce stress.

Most allergists tell you that emotional reactions in and of themselves do not cause asthma, but they do provoke rapid, shallow breathing which prompts the twitchy airways to go into spasm.

The individual (adult or child) can counteract hyperventilation by following these steps:

1. Sit upright in a quiet place. Turn your chair so that you have nothing but the wall to look at.
2. Relax by slumping. Let your neck and shoulders droop loosely.
3. Take slow, deliberate, deep breaths. Inhale through the nose and exhale *slowly* through the mouth. Compress or purse your lips when you exhale to build up back pressure in the airways and keep them open.
4. Continue this for a short period of time. Usually no more than five minutes should be enough to restore the ordinary breathing rhythm and reverse the bronchospasm.
5. Stay relaxed and continue to breathe slowly and deliberately.

AVOIDING ASTHMA-CAUSING DRUGS AND CHEMICALS

Drugs

Drugs can be a dangerous complication in the life of asthmatics.

Louis, 54, has had exercise-induced asthma since childhood. A few months ago he started having chest pains. He went to his doctor for a checkup and was found to have angina, or coronary artery disease. The doctor prescibed propranolol (Inderal) to reduce the severity of the chest pains.

Within hours of taking his first dose of propranolol, Louis began wheezing and his chest tightened and started to heave. Fearing he was having a heart attack, he went to the emergency room; the doctors there hospitalized him, administered oxygen, fed him intravenously, and connected him to the usual electronic monitoring devices. They all read "normal" and one of the doctors, puzzling over the case, guessed that Louis's symptoms might be due to the propranolol. She knew that propranolol, along with other heart medications, can increase the level of muscle tone in the airways, especially in asthmatics.

That proved to be the case for Louis. Fortunately an effective alternative medication was found for him.

Louis learned what every asthmatic should know and practice religiously. Any time you see a doctor or dentist or get a prescription, remind him or her *without fail* that you are asthmatic.

There are three major classes of drugs which are harmful to patients with asthma. These include sedatives, aspirin-like drugs, and drugs that block beta receptors.

Beta blocking drugs are usually given for recurring chest paints, heart disease, and hypertension, or high blood pressure. There are several of these drugs available now, and more are to be released in the next few years. Examples of these drugs are Blocadren, Corgard, Corzide, Inderal, Inderide, Lopressor, Tenoretic, Tenormin, Timolide, and Visken. Be aware that if you are taking beta blocking drugs, some metered aerosols commonly prescribed for asthma, such as Alupent and Ventolin, will *not* work. (See Chapter 15 for more information on beta receptors or agonists.)

A second class of drugs to avoid scrupulously is sedatives or tranquilizers such as Librium, Valium, Vistaril, Thorazine, and all barbiturates. Although asthma often produces anxiety, the anxiety should *never* be treated with tranquilizers. *A common cause of death in patients with asthma is the previous administration of sedative agents to control anxiety.* Sedatives and tranquilizers diminish your respiratory reserve and reduce your breathing capacity. If your doctor prescribes sedatives or tranquilizers, knowing you are asthmatic, it is time to find yourself another doctor *immediately*.

A large number of patients with asthma, perhaps as many as 50–60 percent, will wheeze whenever they take aspirin, ibuprofen (brand names: Motrin, Advil, Nuprin, etc.), or other nonsteroidal anti-inflammatory drugs. In many cases the wheezing is not evident to you and can only be proven when you have pulmonary function testing. This may suggest to you that it is unimportant. However, suppose you have a cold with some diminished respiratory reserve. If you then take aspirin or other nonsteroidal anti-inflammatory drugs, the small amount of effect it has may push you over the edge and into the emergency room. Because of this and other reactions connected with these drugs, we prefer to use acetaminophen (Tylenol, Datril, etc.), which does not aggravate or intensify asthma symptoms.

If you have arthritis or another condition that requires the use of nonsteroidal anti-inflammatory drugs, it is important for your doctor to "challenge" you with these drugs or find a safe alternative. The challenge is done by having you first take a pulmonary function test. You then take the drug by mouth and the pulmonary function testing is repeated 20 minutes, one hour, two hours, and sometimes four hours later. Comparing your pulmonary function values before and after will tell you and your doctor if these drugs are potentially dangerous for you.

DO NOT take any drug without first letting your doctor know about your asthmatic condition. Consult the *Physician's Desk Reference* (available in libraries or the doctor's office) about possible side effects. If even a possibility of an asthmatic reaction is mentioned, do not take the drug. Ask your doctor to provide an alternative medication.

Chemicals

The best-understood cause of chemically induced asthma is sodium meta-bisulfite, a preservative. However, many other preservatives and a rainbow of coloring agents are added to foods. Hundreds of food dyes are in use, and there has been very little research on their safety. Some experts believe that sensitivity to the dye called tartrazine may be a major cause; others say its dangers are exaggerated. We believe that many of these chemicals may be harmful to asthmatics.

Carol's asthma gets worse whenever she ingests foods containing food and dye color #5. Junk food is laced with this chemical, tartrazine — fast-food taco places dish it out by the barrel!

Although Carol scrupulously avoided these foods, she still had problems with her asthma. She was taking the medication prescribed by her doctor and she did not know of any other triggers. Yet she continued to wheeze most of the time. Often her wheezing seemed to get worse after she took her medicine. She mentioned this to her doctor, who discovered that her particular theophylline prescription, one of the most common drugs to treat asthma, contained tartrazine to make it appear more palatable. Carol switched brands and got better.

Fortunately, companies that market asthma drugs have learned from such cases not to put food dyes in asthma remedies. However, antibiotics, birth control pills, hormones, and virtually every other medication do contain food dyes. Whenever you start to take *any* new medication, monitor it carefully to see if it induces your asthma symptoms.

AVOIDING POLLUTION (ESPECIALLY TOBACCO)

The most common and serious of the *air pollutants* is tobacco smoke. ASTHMATICS AND MEMBERS OF THEIR HOUSEHOLD SHOULD NOT SMOKE TOBACCO.

Asthmatics have known for 50 years that tobacco smoke makes them worse, but the influence of tobacco and cigarette smoking on lung and heart disease has come to light only recently. For asthmatics, tobacco has additional sinister implications.

Tobacco smoke is basically a poison gas, which paralyzes the lining of the air tubes and prevents them from clearing out normal mucus and the debris that accumulates every day in lungs. The uncleared mucus becomes extremely thick and may be infected after contact with tobacco smoke. The smoke contains carbon monoxide, which may cause significant pulmonary irritation and can even cause the lungs to collapse. The irritation it causes makes your fragile air sacs even weaker and more vulnerable.

In addition to the effects of smoking yourself, considerable attention has been focused on the role of secondhand smoke produced by smokers in your home, office, restaurants, on international airline flights, and so forth. Secondhand smoke definitely has the potential to irritate asthmatic lungs. A number of studies have shown that children who reside in homes where parents smoke have more frequent and longer hospitalizations for asthma than do children who live in nonsmoking environments.

Everyone has the right to breathe clean air. As an asthmatic, you should not be exposed to anything that could adversely affect your health. There are a number of things asthmatics can do about tobacco smoke:

- Declare your home a No-Smoking Zone.
- Discuss your need for smoke-free air with your co-workers. You may be surprised to find how readily people will alter their smoking habit when they learn the nature of your health problems.
- Always seek out smoke-free areas in public places. Ask for nonsmokers' rooms in hotels.

Bill has had asthma for approximately 15 years. As he has gotten older, his asthma has become a bit more difficult to treat. He suspects the reason is that he is now driving to work on smog-congested freeways. Moreover, he works in a busy office where 6 out of 13 people smoke constantly. At first he was very irritated with the smokers and asked them to stop smoking. All that did was create friction. About three weeks ago an acute asthma attack had him hospitalized for four days in the Intensive Care Unit at a local hospital. When he returned to work he discussed it with his boss. The co-workers got together and discussed it amongst themselves. Bill was very gratified to find out how supportive they were. Smoking is now allowed in the hallway and in the coffee room of the office. All other places in the office have been declared nonsmoking. Bill's asthma is still a problem but he does feel better and thinks he has been able to reduce at least this trigger.

Stopping smoking, for someone with a well-established habit, is extraordinarily difficult. There are a variety of programs designed to help smokers kick the tobacco habit. None of them is 100 percent effective, but the best ones are those that are conducted by a local respiratory society or that apply behavioral modification techniques to overcome the addiction. Your local Lung or Heart Association as well as local hospitals will know of and be able to refer you to programs aimed at stopping smoking.

High concentrations of ozone and sulfur dioxide — air pollution — are a potent cause of asthma. They are the result of a conspiracy of climatic conditions and automobile emissions which cause asthmatics considerable distress.

Most cities with significant smog problems forecast air quality in the morning newspaper. If the smog index is "high" or "alert," then it is especially dangerous for asthmatics, because the pollutant indexes relate to normal people. Thus people with respiratory disease will start showing symptoms when the index is "moderate." When that happens, or is about to happen, remain indoors. Keep your windows closed and relax. Do not go out until the smog clears. If you must go out, wear a disposable paper mask, much like the ones worn by surgeons and carpenters, which are available at any drugstore. The mask will not lower the level of sulfur dioxide or other gaseous pollutants but will filter out some particulate matter. When you go out, do not exercise or otherwise exert yourself. Walk at a moderate pace and avoid other obvious triggering factors in the environment like automobile emissions and tobacco smoke.

OTHER TRIGGERS

There are a myriad of other substances we have not discussed that are capable of causing an asthmatic reaction. Many household cleaning products, especially detergents and aerosol cleaners, can set you to wheezing; so can solvents, glues, cosmetics, perfumes, and powders. Exposure to feathers or goose down in comforters or sleeping bags can cause trouble, as can smoke from a fireplace or candles or fumes from kerosene lamps.

In all of these instances, detection is relatively easy (see Chapter 5) and avoidance is equally straightforward and simple. There are nonallergenic substitutes available for all of them, save for the candles on the birthday cake. Use one symbolic candle and remove it as soon as it has been blown out — not as much fun, perhaps, but better than a bronchospasm.

RELOCATION

Relocating is the ultimate avoidance tactic. Years ago, before many of the medications now available for the treatment of asthma were discovered, it was often recommended that sufferers move to a warm, dry climate. Arizona and New Mexico were commonly suggested.

It may be that this sort of advice was fueled by anecdotes of patients whose asthma — or allergies generally — improved significantly on relocation. And, in some instances, where the cause was definitely established and could be totally avoided by relocating, such moves did work. However, there is no evidence that the population of the Southwest is significantly freer of allergic disease than those who live in harsher climates. Uprooting and moving a family to another location to escape asthma or other allergic disease is a hazardous and often crushingly disappointing step. It is more sensible — and no less successful — to take determined steps to control asthma in the home territory.

Diet and Asthma

REACTIONS TO FOOD: ALLERGY OR SENSITIVITY?

Virtually any food or drink can trigger an asthmatic reaction in a susceptible person. In some instances the asthmatic symptoms represent a true
allergic (atopic or IgE related) response; in most cases the reaction is not
a true allergy but merely an intolerance or hypersensitivity. The difference
is important in that it may distinguish potentially life-threatening reactions
from minor inconveniences.

A wide variety of foods, food colors, and food preservatives, or pre-
existing conditions in the individual, can also produce symptoms that
closely mimic asthmatic reactions and, in fact, account for most negative
reactions to "food." This mimicry makes precise diagnosis extremely difficult. However, there is considerable comfort in the knowledge that, while
diagnosis of the reasons for food intolerances is complicated and uncertain,
treatment of your food hypersensitivity (as we prefer to call it) is extremely
easy — simply stay away from whatever is causing your problem. Whether
the reaction is truly allergic or not isn't necessarily as important as finding
out what is doing the mischief and steering clear of it.

As we noted in Chapter 1, an asthmatic reaction is a bodily defense (the
immune system) gone wrong. When we are exposed to germs and foreign
substances we ordinarily make antibodies. If our food were to be injected
directly into the body (most foods are foreign to the body) we would
routinely produce antibodies to repel the invader. However, food is eaten,
not injected; it is digested in the stomach, where it is degraded into fine
chemical units that are readily accepted by our bodies. (In very young
children, and in some older people, undigested quantities of food some-

times do get absorbed; this may be the reason for increased problems with food-related asthma in these age groups.)

It is often difficult to establish whether an asthmatic reaction to food represents a true allergic reaction. Even allergists disagree on the definition of what constitutes a food allergy. The more cautious ones limit the diagnosis of food-linked asthma to those instances where tests detect the presence of the antibody IgE. Others believe that, when the classic asthmatic symptoms — wheezing, shortness of breath, mucus production — are present, the diagnosis of allergic or atopic asthma is probably accurate, even if no antibody is found. To the sufferers the symptoms are the same, and to keep symptom-free they should avoid the offending agent.

THE USUAL COURSE OF A HYPERSENSITIVE ASTHMATIC REACTION TO FOOD

Food hypersensitivity can be expressed as wheezing and shortness of breath. However, there is no "usual" course, and symptoms can vary dramatically in their severity. (See Tables 4 and 5.) What happens depends on a host of factors, including the degree of sensitivity or vulner-

TABLE 4   Symptoms of Food Hypersensitivity

Location of Reaction	Children	Adults
Gastrointestinal	Colic, vomiting, diarrhea	Diarrhea, cramps, constipation
Pulmonary	Wheezing, shortness of breath, cough	Wheezing, shortness of breath
Ear, nose, and throat	Runny nose, nasal congestion, ear inflammation	Runny nose, nasal congestion
Central nervous system	Headache	Headache
Skin	Eczema, hives, itching	Eczema, hives, itching
Vascular	Faintness, drop in blood pressure, loss of consciousness (rare in infants)	Faintness, drop in blood pressure, loss of consciousness
Psychological	Irritability, hyperactivity*	Irritability, depression, psychosis
Other		Tension-fatigue syndrome

*Hyperactivity or hyperkinesis: despite widespread popular belief to the contrary, there is little credible evidence linking this troublesome syndrome to particular foods.

Type of Reaction	Symptoms
1. Anaphylactic (within seconds to 30 minutes)	Pallor, shock, intense and widespread itchiness, wheezing, shortness of breath, hives
2. Immediate (3 to 60 minutes)	Vomiting, diarrhea, wheezing, shortness of breath, itching, hives
3. Intermediate (1 to 12 hours)	Vomiting, diarrhea, hives, wheezing, shortness of breath, nasal congestion or runniness, flaring of eczema, headache, cough
4. Delayed* (after 12 hours)	Tension-fatigue syndrome, "allergic" manifestations, respiratory discomfort, depression

*With the exception of conditions resulting from gastrointestinal disorders, which are tied to malabsorption of food, the evidence for delayed hypersensitive reactions is largely anecdotal and not backed by hard, scientific data.

ability of the individual and the amount and form in which the irritant is ingested. There are instances when an asthmatic reaction to food is unbelievably swift and severe.

Kim, a 17-year-old girl, is staying overnight with a group of her girlfriends. She prepares a snack for herself: a tuna fish sandwich and soda. After a few minutes she complains that she doesn't feel well, breaks out in hives, starts having severe breathing difficulties, becomes confused, and comes close to passing out. The parents of the hostess rush her to the emergency room of a nearby hospital where she is treated for anaphylaxis (or an acute allergic reaction). Fortunately, Kim recovers quickly. It turns out that Kim is violently allergic to peanuts. Kim knows that and scrupulously avoids contact with peanuts or foods containing peanuts. What she did not know is that the knife that she picked up and used to make her sandwich contained a small amount of peanut butter left by its previous user — a microscopic quantity, but enough to produce Kim's near-fatal reaction.

In most instances, happily, the sequence of events is more leisurely and the symptoms less grave.

MEDICAL EVALUATION FOR FOOD-HYPERSENSITIVE ASTHMATIC REACTIONS

Sometimes identifying an asthmatic reaction to a particular food or substance is no problem at all and a doctor is not necessary.

For years Ted had followed the custom of having a glass of robust red wine with dinner. Just about the time he turned 60 he began having a dull, throbbing headache and a slight wheeze most evenings. He had his blood pressure checked but that seemed to be fine. He didn't have any other problems and during the day at work he felt well. Then he went on a pack trip with a couple of friends and didn't have anything alcoholic to drink for three days. No headaches or shortness of breath either. When he got home from the camping trip he followed the simple expedient of drinking, as usual, some nights, and not drinking other nights, and recording his reaction. The results were invariant — if he drank he had a headache and a wheeze, but with no alcohol he had no symptoms.

It is probably safe not to see a doctor when the offending food is positively identified; it does not provoke a life-threatening reaction; it is easily and successfully avoided; and not consuming the food leads to a complete remission of symptoms. In all other cases, seek medical advice to get help in establishing what is causing your problem and in developing effective ways to deal with it. This is especially true because some instances of what appear to be food intolerance are actually manifestations of organic deficiencies or chronic illnesses. If not recognized and treated appropriately these conditions can threaten life. And, in the case of anaphylactic reactions, medical advice is absolutely necessary to devise comprehensive avoidance strategies and to develop familiarity with and competence in administering emergency procedures.

THE LEADING CAUSES OF ASTHMATIC REACTIONS TO FOOD

Any food — and many of the substances found in it or added to it to enhance its appearance or growth, ward off insects, improve its flavor, preserve its freshness — is capable of setting off a reaction in a susceptible person. The condition or state of the individual — illness, enzyme deficiencies, thyroid malfunctions — can also interact with foods to cause reactions.

The foods that appear on any list of leading causes of food hypersensitivity depend on the expert doing the listing. There is agreement that cow's milk, eggs, shellfish, nuts, and wheat provoke reactions, but the unanimity stops there. Legumes (peanuts and soybeans) are frequently mentioned, as are fish and mollusks. However, authorities disagree on the role of tomatoes, chocolate, and citrus fruits, which are popularly identified as *allergens*, although strict laboratory experiments fail to support this charge. (Chocolate can make you sick, but it is not borne out that the sickness is allergic.) The nomination of other substances like cola apparently owes as much to subjective bias as to scientific study.

To make matters more confusing, certain foods like strawberries, other berries, and tomatoes, which certainly cause rashes, especially in young children, are often deemed allergens by parents. In fact, there is no evidence at all that "strawberry rash" is IgE mediated. Some people are hypersensitive to strawberries but not "allergic" to them. Table 6 illustrates the wide range of symptoms that foods and additives can induce.

TABLE 6 Causes of Intolerance and Characteristic Symptoms

Causal Agent	Symptoms
Foods such as strawberries, tomatoes, citrus fruits, shellfish	Rash, itching
Mold that is often found in cheeses, fermented meats like salami, fermented beverages like beer, dried fruits, yogurt	Rash, itching, respiratory problems
Antibiotic contaminants (bacitracin, penicillin, tetracycline) found in meats, poultry, or milk	Rash, itching, respiratory, gastrointestinal (GI) problems
Insect residues in spices	Rash, itching, respiratory, GI problems
Chemical food additives Monosodium glutamate (MSG)	"Chinese restaurant syndrome" (flushing, headache, chest pain)
Metabisulfite, tartrazine	GI symptoms, headache, rash, itching, respiratory problems
Bacteria and bacterial toxins	GI symptoms — pain, gas, diarrhea
Enzyme deficiencies	GI symptoms, colic (in infants)
GI tract diseases including gastric and duodenal ulcers, hiatal hernia	Gastric distress (pain, burning, gas)

IDENTIFYING THE CAUSES OF FOOD-RELATED ASTHMA

Earlier we drew attention to the fact that there is little agreement about what a "food allergy" is or what brings it on. This is why the study and treatment of food intolerance is one of the most difficult areas in the whole field of clinical allergy. Identifying the cause of a reaction and developing successful tactics for avoiding it, although tricky, can be accomplished if you pay close attention to your symptoms and keep careful records.

A strategy to follow in identifying the food (or the myriad of additives, contaminants, or other conditions) responsible for a hypersensitive asthmatic reaction is sketched in Figure 6. The figure outlines what is essentially a conservative, and minimally risky, series of steps to follow in finding out the cause of your hypersensitive reaction to food. *The key to finding out*

FIGURE 6   Identifying Food Hypersensitivity

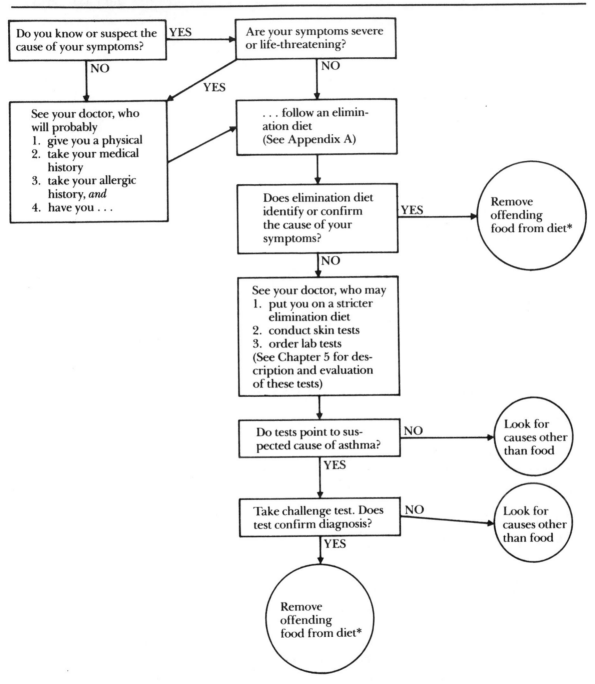

*See Appendixes B, C, and D for dye- and chemical-free diets. Foods by themselves rarely trigger asthma.

the information you need is careful observance of an elimination diet. (A general elimination diet, together with the steps you will need to follow to see it through to a successful conclusion, is presented in Appendix A.) Following the procedures outlined in Figure 6 and sticking faithfully to the elimination diet, if it is called for, should point to whatever is causing your wheezes. The hardest part of the process may be to force yourself to stay on the diet, which can be monotonous.

When you do isolate the source of your reaction, your problems are over — almost. Along the way, however, there are a few things to know and to be careful about.

- *Do not* allow skin tests or challenges if your food intolerance is severe or life-threatening.
- *Challenge tests* are the key to dead-sure identification of specific causes of food hypersensitivity. If done, they should be conducted "double-blind" so that neither you nor the person giving the test knows if the offending substance or a non–symptom-producing "placebo" is being served up. In a double-blind challenge test, your doctor prepares a number of gelatin capsules. Some capsules are filled with glucose (sugar). Others are filled with different quantities of the suspected food. The capsules are mixed up so that neither you nor your doctor knows what is in there, although they are coded so that they can be identified later. Your reactions to each capsule you take are recorded, and the record becomes the basis for deciding whether or not you are hypersensitive to the food with which you are being challenged.
- *A justly suspected food may not lead to a reaction,* when tested, because of the method of preparation, the amount consumed, the presence of other foods, or the state of the sample. If you have a good circumstantial case against a particular suspect, do not give up testing it too quickly.
- *Skin tests* (scratch or prick) for food hypersensitivity are crude, cover only a small fraction of the possibilities, are potentially dangerous, and are useful mainly in their ability to identify *lack* of sensitivity to a substance. They will rule out potential offenders — but the potential offenders, alas, far outnumber the specific tests available. A course of skin testing will likely eliminate some suspects, turn up a few false leads (false positive reactions), and, if you are very lucky, the real culprit.

The Role of Food in Individuals with Multiple Allergies

Many allergy sufferers produce high levels of IgE to a number, sometimes a multitude, of foreign proteins. They may display allergic symptoms ranging from hay fever to asthma, plus watery eyes, chest congestion, and skin reactions. Are these symptoms due entirely to things in the air, such as pollens, dust, or animal dander? Some of them may also be partially ascribed to food. It is difficult to know when food is implicated, because in such individuals food sensitivity may be an element in but not the entire problem. In these cases reliance on the history and looking for a seasonal pattern of symptoms is extremely important; faithfully keeping the ASTHMA FINDER (Figure 5 in Chapter 5) is therefore vital. Do your symptoms get worse certain seasons of the year? Are they worse after meals? Do they occur more or less frequently when traveling or eating away from home?

There are also some special associations in people who have hay fever and coincidental sensitivity to certain foods. Some individuals with hay fever develop severe itching of the mouth, swelling of the throat, and breathing problems when they eat peaches, avocados, or melons. These reactions show up primarily during the hay fever season; at other times the problems these foods produce are minimal.

Another special problem with multiple allergies occurs in children. Children often absorb small quantities of food that remain undigested. The body recognizes these undigested foods as foreign, makes IgE antibodies, and food allergy appears. As children grow older, however, their gastrointestinal tracts mature, food is digested completely, and absorption of small quantities of undigested food no longer occurs. With this maturation of the intestine and proper food digestion, the symptoms of food allergy generally disappear. However, if these children later develop pollen sensitivity their food allergies may return.

Mysterious Hidden Food Allergies

The fact that some individuals have a variety of nonspecific complaints, such as tension fatigue and headache, associated with food, and the fact that it is very difficult to diagnose food allergy using blood or skin tests has made the entire subject of food sensitivity a hotbed of controversy. Many people (and many physicians too) wrongly believe that it is impossible to make a firm diagnosis of food allergy. Rather, they contend that some hidden insidious sensitivity to food causes a form of asthma (and/or hay fever or eczema) that responds to treatment poorly. This view of the role of food in asthma is not correct and has never been borne out by rigorous scientific testing. Given a proper history, a carefully kept diary, and appropriate laboratory tests, your physician should be quite capable of determining exactly what foods you cannot tolerate and what part they play in your symptoms.

Nonallergic Asthmatic Reactions to Foods

As we have said, the diagnosis of a *true* allergy requires the presence of IgE, which binds onto special white cells known as basophils or mast cells and — under appropriate circumstances (such as eating the food you are allergic to) — causes them to release histamine and the other chemicals that set you to wheezing. However, there are ways that allergens can directly cause your white cells to release histamine and the chemicals without IgE involvement. A large number of foods and drugs are capable of doing this. The best example is sensitivity to berries, and strawberries in particular, in children. Sensitive children, if they eat berries, may develop itching, hives, breathing problems, or even a full-blown anaphylactic reaction. This sensitivity to berries often disappears as the child gets older.

Another, perhaps better known syndrome is "allergy" to shrimp, clams, oysters, lobster, or other crustaceans. The symptoms of only a small number can be linked to IgE.

> Vickie has enjoyed good health all of her life but notes that after eating shrimp she breaks out in hives and, if she gets enough of them, wheezes too. She carefully avoids eating shrimp at home. However, as part of Vickie's job she is often called upon to appear at meetings and banquets. She has found that a large number of hors d'oeuvres contain small minces of shrimp. Vickie has encountered shrimp stuffed in mushrooms or tomatoes, camouflaged in dips or mixed in large Caesar salads, and everywhere in Chinese and Japanese restaurants. She even reacts if the pan used to cook her dinner previously contained shrimp. Since she is often called on to speak — and her reaction to shrimp affects her dramatically — she has learned to carry an antihistamine in her purse. Even when she does not suspect that shrimp is on the menu, as a precaution she takes an antihistamine about 20 minutes before dinner. This prevents her from developing symptoms unless she inadvertently consumes large quantities of shellfish.

Much like those with childhood sensitivity to strawberries, these individuals experience the direct release of histamine and chemicals from their basophils or mast cells without having any IgE. Thus, according to a strict medical definition, they do not have an allergy to these foods. However, the end result is exactly the same, and they may develop anything from minor wheezing to swelling of the throat and anaphylaxis. Unlike allergy to berries, however, the reaction to crustaceans does not tend to go away in adults.

The greatest offender of all in these peculiar non-IgE reactions are food dyes and preservatives. Prominent among these triggers is tartrazine, the yellow food dye found in tacos, potato chips, capsules of medicine, some toothpastes, and hundreds of other products. Persons who are hypersensitive to tartrazine are often sensitive to aspirin too. These aspirin-susceptible persons often develop asthma or have their asthma worsen if they eat foods containing tartrazine. (See Appendix B.)

Controlling Asthmatic Symptoms
Caused by Food Intolerance

Avoidance is the safest and most effective tactic to follow in controlling asthmatic symptoms due to food intolerance. If complete avoidance is not possible (because the list of irritants is long and diffuse), and if the hypersensitivity is truly immunological or allergic, then suppressing symptoms through medication is sometimes a workable alternative. *This control step should be taken only under medical supervision.*

Sometimes recurring reactions are due to lack of willpower.

> Bob is truly hypersensitive to chocolate and whenever he eats it he immediately slips into an attack of allergic rhinitis — a streaming nose and a nasty postnasal drip — with some minor asthmatic symptoms. Yet, despite the acute discomfort it causes him, he has never succeeded in putting aside his craving for chocolate. Whenever he yields to the temptation to eat a candy bar he follows it with an Allerest chaser. He knows he would be better off if he never ate chocolate again, but admits he lacks the self-discipline to do so.

DIET RECOMMENDATIONS

There are a few fad diets and any number of home remedies or patent medicines that claim to relieve asthma. None of them has been proved effective in practice or has stood scientific testing, and some of them (nasal drops or sprays, for example) can actually make matters worse.

On the other hand, a strong case can be made for the importance of a well-rounded diet in the prevention of asthma. Any time you become weak and run-down because of a vitamin-deficient, unbalanced junk food–dominated diet, you are setting yourself up for infections. Since colds and infections are the most important asthma-triggering agents, a poor diet can contribute directly to more frequent and more severe asthmatic attacks.

Common sense is the guideline. Get enough foods in the major food groups to satisfy recommended minimum daily requirements for proteins, carbohydrates, fats, vitamins, and minerals. Avoid excesses, particularly of stimulants, salt, sugar, and alcohol (not more than 1½ ounces daily — two 12-ounce cans of beer or two light cocktails or three 4-ounce glasses of wine). Limit consumption of red meats (once every other day is plenty) and eat plenty of fresh fruits and vegetables, cooked or (preferably) raw. Wash fresh vegetables and fruits carefully even if they are advertised as completely organic. (Foods described as "natural" may still contain preservatives and chemicals; read the list of ingredients carefully.) Drink plenty of liquids and provide for some fiber either through breads, vegetable intake, or cereal brans. Do not overeat and after eating take a few minutes before you resume stressful activities. A brief nap after lunch can work wonders. Depending on your ability to tolerate it, be judicious in your use of milk and milk products — cheese, cottage cheese, ice cream, yogurt, etc. Avoid "empty calorie" foods such as snack foods, which provide calories but no other food value. Limit the number of heavily salted, high fat, fried "fast foods." Eat at regular times and try not to eat "on the go." Provide adequate time to sit down and enjoy your meal.

It is important not to use food as a lever or bribe for an asthmatic child. All too often a worried parent will try to coax a child into acting better by fixing favorite dishes; this tactic can promote or encourage the appearance — or the claim — of symptoms.

Foods to Relieve Asthma Symptoms

It has been known for a long time that hot black coffee will make breathing easier, relieve wheezing, and help in mucus production. If you are having a mild bout with asthma, coffee may help, but should not be considered a replacement for medication.

It also helps to drink large quantities of fluids, for two reasons:

1. The labored mouth-breathing so characteristic of an asthma attack has the effect of expelling much more moisture and may lead to dehydration.
2. A proper liquid balance is essential to raising and getting rid of airway-blocking mucus.

Water is probably the best and safest liquid to drink, although "sports drinks" are sometimes recommended. Formulated to imitate the chemical composition of body fluid, they are thought to be more easily assimilated by the body.

Because they may contribute to an asthmatic reaction, certain liquids should probably be avoided: orange or other citrus juices, milk, chocolate milk, and soft drinks and punches that contain preservatives or food dyes. Anecdotal evidence claims that chicken soup laced with garlic helps asthmatics, but, unfortunately, the evidence is not credible. Apart from coffee (hot or cold) and other beverages containing significant amounts of caffeine, no food or drink has proved to ease the symptoms of asthma.

CHAPTER 8

Chemical and Occupational Asthma

It has been known for more than 250 years that asthma may be caused by materials other than pollens, animal danders, and house dust. In 1713 an Italian physician named Ramazzini described asthmalike symptoms occurring in men who worked in flour mills. Ramazzini believed the coughing and wheezing these men suffered was due to a reaction between the grain and their lungs. Since then, chemicals have literally saturated the workplace, the home, and the environment. Chemicals not only are more sophisticated but also have multiplied ten thousand-fold in the last century. It is impossible to avoid exposure to chemicals: our clothes, our food, the air we breathe are all contaminated with them. We do not imply that exposure to chemicals always makes asthmatics worse; however, many chemicals can produce allergic and asthmatic reactions, and thousands of others can cause nonallergic sensitivity reactions.

There are three ways chemical sensitivity can make asthma worse:

1. Exposure to some chemicals, like toluene, stimulates the production of IgE, which can cause asthma.
2. Other chemicals, like IVP (the dye used to take kidney X rays), can cause body mast cells or white cells to degranulate and release histamine directly, even without IgE. Chemicals and drugs having this tendency include codeine and polymyxin.
3. Some chemicals are such harsh irritants that they can make your bronchial muscles go into spasm. Prominent among these irritants are plastics, gasoline fumes, and some glues.

REACTIONS TO CHEMICALS: ALLERGY OR SENSITIVITY?

A true allergy, as we have noted, is a reaction mediated by the antibody immunoglobulin E. There are other types of reactions occurring in many people that some physicians interpret as allergic, when in fact they represent sensitivity. The difference between allergy and sensitivity is an important one.

> Peter and Sam have been partners in a house painting business for nearly 15 years. Peter has always maintained that he likes the smell of fresh paint, even though he knows that the fumes and the paint itself contain chemicals. Sam, on the other hand, has always hated the smell of paint. Almost from the very beginning he developed nausea and headaches whenever exposed to paint. He continued to work as a painter despite these complaints. Recently, his headaches and nausea have gotten worse and he has also developed dizzy spells. Medical tests showed that Sam does not have a true allergy to paint; yet it is quite clear that his symptoms are real and that he is very sensitive to its fumes. His doctor advised him to give up house painting and find other work. Sam believed that the only way he could give up painting was to have his condition diagnosed as an allergy, thus qualifying him for disability.

There are many other materials with strong odors that make people develop nausea, giddiness, or headaches. Most of these materials will not produce asthma, but certain ones, if they show up in the air you breathe, do have the potential to trigger asthma or to make it worse without any allergic (IgE) involvement.

Particulate matter and smog provoke chemical sensitivities and, along with sulfur dioxide and ozone in the air, aggravate asthmatic symptoms by increasing the twitchiness of airways. Strong odors can also make asthma get worse in this same way. Table 7 lists odor-producing substances or materials that can have this effect.

TABLE 7   Sources of Asthma-Provoking Odors or Fumes

aerosols	formaldehyde (formalin)
alcohol (rubbing)	incense
ammonia	ink
bubble bath or oils	insect repellents
camphor	moth balls
candles	paints
castor beans (flour or oil)	perfumes
cleaning fluid	phenol
coal, gasoline, kerosene, oil	polyurethane
cosmetics	smoke
creosote	soaps
deodorants	tobacco
detergents	toluene
floor wax	turpentine

OCCUPATIONAL ASTHMA

There are a myriad of materials found in the workplace that have the potential to make asthma and allergies worse. The symptoms may include everything from hay fever with sneezing, nasal congestion, runny nose, watery eyes, and hives to asthma. Table 8 lists industries that use these materials.

The histories of individuals having occupational asthma are often very similar to Joe's:

> Joe shows up for work Monday morning at 8:00 feeling great. He gets off work about 5:00 and stops off at a local bar for a beer on his way home. At 8:00 P.M., so punctually that Joe can set his watch by it, he begins to cough and wheeze. He coughs and wheezes throughout the evening and almost into the night, relieved only by medication. By morning he is fine and goes back to work.
>
> At first Joe's doctor thought that Joe might be allergic to beer or something at home. Despite numerous tests they could not find the probable cause. Moreover, Joe pointed out that nothing ailed him at home on weekends. His doctor then concluded that something on the job was bothering Joe. Joe worked in a processing plant that converted whole to powdered milk. Joe explained that he loathes milk and he doesn't even eat ice cream because it gives him diarrhea.
>
> The doctor, intrigued, had Joe avoid all milk products for a few days and then drink a glass of milk. Nothing happened. The doctor concluded Joe was not allergic to milk, but asked Joe whether there are fumes or odors of powdered milk at work. "Everywhere," Joe replied.
>
> Joe was referred to an allergist who found Joe had high levels of antibody directed at milk proteins. He also had Joe inhale a very small quantity of powdered milk. Four hours after the inhalation challenge test, Joe began to wheeze.

This delayed daily reaction, with asthma developing several hours after work, is typical of what occurs in many individuals who have occupational asthma. Other patterns include progressive deterioration during the week,

TABLE 8 Industries Linked to Chemically Induced Asthma

Communications and electronics
Detergent manufacturing or distribution
Dyeing and photocopying
Food production, processing, and packaging
Lacquer and rubber manufacturing
Metal refining and plating
Oil production, refining, or distribution
Paint, plastics, and coatings, especially ones using polyurethane
Pharmaceuticals and drugs
Printing
Textile weaving or finishing (natural or synthetic fabrics)

with the worker rebounding over the weekend, or sometimes a gradual decline week by week, in pulmonary function.

Specific Causes of Occupational Asthma

People who are sensitive (or allergic) to wheat, rye, or other flours suffer from what has long been called "baker's asthma." Dust from coffee or castor beans can also be a problem, even affecting people who live near plants that disperse these materials into the air. Asthma has been noted frequently in occupations that entail exposure to trimellitic anhydride (used in making plastics, epoxy resins, and paints) or isocyanide (involved in producing polyurethane insulation, paint, and adhesives). Formaldehyde, which can appear in plywood, insulation, wallpaper, carpeting, furniture, and other products associated with the building industry, is a major trigger of asthma. The symptoms it provokes are acute, a direct and immediate response to the insult offered by the chemical itself, and they should disappear after one leaves the contaminated environment. In addition, asthma has turned up in individuals who work in "tight" office buildings.

Do You Have Occupational Asthma?

The procedures to follow in determining if you have occupational asthma are essentially the same as those used in nailing down other causes for the appearance of the disease. (See Chapter 5.) First, maintain a careful record or history of the onset of the attacks and their relationship to other activities in your life. Then if you suspect occupational asthma consult a physician, either your own doctor or, if it has one, the company's. The doctor should help you determine if your asthma results directly from exposure to substances you encounter at work or is due to other reasons. In the case of hard-to-diagnose symptoms, you may be in for a long series of tests, which would include a good physical examination and skin testing, particularly effective in spotting asthma caused by trimellitic anhydride, coffee beans, and enzymes or detergents. Pulmonary function tests in the workplace before and after exposure to potentially triggering substances may be conducted, and a laboratory-based series of inhalation challenge tests may also be carried out. This last should be done only if the suspected agent can be accurately measured and administered in dosages below the acute irritant level and if there are no contraindications like heart disease. If carried out, a physician should be present because, as with all respiratory challenges, there is an element of serious risk. Such tests require a preliminary period of preparation, and the actual tests may extend over a period of up to six days.

Hypersensitivity Pneumonitis and Occupational Asthma

If something on your job provokes persistent, recurring asthma, even mild, you have only one recourse — avoid the insult and immediately remove yourself from that workplace. Continued exposure can make the asthma much worse and may lead to the development of a serious syndrome called hypersensitivity pneumonitis.

This condition, most often resulting from exposure to agents encountered at work, is a distant cousin of asthma. People with it virtually always display sensitivity or allergy to chemicals or airborne allergens generally found in specific occupations. They may include farmers allergic to moldy hay, office workers sensitive to mold growing in office air conditioners, or lumber mill workers sensitive to redwood or maple dust. In addition to wheezing, these people develop an inflammation in the lung itself, which, if unchecked, leads to severe lung damage. Table 9 lists a few of the more common known causes and occupations that are associated with this relatively rare type of lung inflammation. If you suspect that something in your work environment is impairing your health, we strongly urge you to seek medical attention and to avoid further exposure on the job until the issue is resolved.

THE TREATMENT OF OCCUPATIONAL ASTHMA

Occupational asthma is treated much like any other asthma. It commonly results from substances entering the respiratory system. If exposure is absolutely unvoidable, reduce the risk with a special face mask, even though it is cumbersome and uncomfortable. Workers who handle chemicals to which they are sensitive often find special hoods helpful.

TABLE 9 **Causes and Conditions Associated with Hypersensitivity Pneumonitis**

Cause	Conditions*
Bacteria (actinomyces) resulting from fermentation of organic matter	Farmer's lung, mushroom worker's lung, fog fever
Molds or fungi	Cheese-maker's lung, humidifier lung, sauna-taker's disease
Dusts or other airborne allergens or contaminants	Bird fancier's lung, wood dust disease, coffee worker's lung, ventilation system pneumonitis

*The list of conditions is illustrative only and not intended to be complete or definitive.

Drug therapy for occupational asthma is the same as that for ordinary asthma. However, medications do carry side effects, which may render the work environment more hazardous; this risk should be kept in mind.

Allergy shots are hardly ever used in individuals with occupational asthma because the allergen or antigen may be unknown, the appropriate dosages (concentrations) have not been worked out, or because they are potentially dangerous. The only exceptions are veterinarians with extreme sensitivity to animal danders.

In some instances the prognosis for occupational asthma may be very poor. A good deal depends on the length and severity of your exposure.

Remember Sam, the house painter we discussed earlier? Sam's symptoms, although not due to IgE and non-diagnosable by conventional tests, are nonetheless real. Sam's body is extremely sensitive to and irritated by chemicals or paint fumes. He cannot totally avoid these chemicals, which are contained in paint as well as floor polishes, the ink in some newspapers, mimeograph machines, and so on. Despite the obviousness of his distress and the clear cause of it, Sam has a hard time convincing anyone that his problem has physical rather than emotional roots. This is often the plight of individuals with occupational asthma and one that needs understanding and clarification.

Environmental Safeguards

The growing prevalence of chemicals in the environment and their ability to provoke asthmatic symptoms have led some physicians and hospitals to devise heroic procedures for providing facilities or environments that are chemically free. These tactics are sometimes recommended for individuals either for whom treatment has proved ineffective or whose reactions are so severe that they cannot live a normal life. The more extreme cases are called "universal reactors" and their condition is sometimes referred to as "twentieth-century disease."

This development in treatment procedures, an outgrowth of the widespread concern with ecological issues, has been enthusiastically adopted by a group of practitioners who refer to themselves as clinical ecologists. Recent observations of this drastic treatment found that most of the individuals studied, who manifested diffuse reactions to toxic chemicals, actually suffered from psychosomatic ailments and that the stringent environmental measures taken to remedy their complaints were ineffectual in almost all cases.

We have no doubt that there are those whose symptoms do ease when they are freed of chemical influences, but there are others whose symptoms would have cleared regardless of steps taken. The complex and virtually unknown relationship between allergic (and asthmatic) complaints and the emotional status of the individual certainly needs further study. Your doctor should be expected to listen carefully to your complaint, be it allergy or sensitivity, and to pull out all the stops in doing what is best for you.

Sports, Exercise, and the Asthmatic

More than three hundred years ago, Sir John Floyer, an eminent British surgeon, wrote "violent exercise makes the asthmatic to breathe short." For years exercise has been recognized as being one of the many factors that can induce bronchospasm or increase twitchiness of airways. In fact, in many, exercise is the *only* obvious asthma-producing trigger. Those children and adults who show asthmatic reactions only to vigorous exercise probably have a predisposition to asthma but fortunately do not have it in its complete form.

THE IMPORTANCE OF EXERCISE

Physical activity maintains both physical and psychological health, especially in children. Daily play is vital to the process of growing up and developing peer interactions and relationships. Children who have asthma, including exercise-induced asthma, must be encouraged and helped to participate in physical activity and training to the fullest extent possible, consistent with health considerations. To do less would be to blunt their maturation, compound problems of low self-esteem, and run the risk of creating other psychosocial problems. Asthma need not control their lives. Physicians treating asthmatic children and parents must formulate specific programs to increase respiratory reserve and condition the child. To this should be added the best pharmacotherapy available to treat the hyperirritable airways. *Avoiding exercise because of asthma is not only unwarranted — it is harmful as well.*

FACTORS IN PREVENTING EXERCISE-INDUCED ASTHMA

Studies clearly show that exercise can induce bronchospasm or asthma in four out of five children with asthma. It can also cause wheezing in many other individuals who do not have asthma. Even so, some of these susceptible children have gone on to become outstanding athletes, even Olympic competitors. There are a number of factors that are important in determining how and how well asthmatics can participate in physical activities and sports.

- Asthmatics are often in poor physical respiratory condition and even a small amount of exercise may be difficult for them and may make their asthma worse.
- However, children with asthma require physical activity much like other children. Moreover, they need to be in *better* shape than other children, so that they have a physical reserve to fall back on when they have problems.
- Children with exercise-associated asthma benefit from a program of endurance training and muscle strengthening exercises. This type of program allows them to increase their exercise tolerance.
- It is essential that asthmatic (and other) children develop a positive attitude toward physical activity and come to enjoy it for its own sake, without feeling awkward or inferior.
- Children want to be part of a group. Too often asthmatic children are relegated to onlooker status, wanting to join in but unable, unwilling, or afraid to do so.
- Children with asthma are often wrongly excused from gym class. A physical training program can be devised to give them the strength and encouragement they need to perform competently in and enjoy physical exercise and team sports. (See Appendix I.)

Scott has had asthma all of his life, his first attack occurring at the age of eight months. His mother noted that virtually anything that changed in Scott's life would induce him to wheeze — changing from formula to milk, going from warm indoor air to the outdoors, excitement, fever. So she was not at all surprised when Scott was asked to sit out routine childhood play activities during nursery school; the teacher commented that even when Scott sang too loudly she would hear wheezing. Scott was kept out of physical activity in school. As Scott grew older his asthma grew much less severe. Nonetheless, he continued to believe and was told that he could not participate in gym. For Scott's entire school career, he was an onlooker. He did not join the Boy Scouts or school clubs, he did not date, he avoided attending sports activities and school events. Despite this his grades were good. His parents were overprotective and constantly reminded him of how serious his asthma had been. Scott is now in college. He has never really learned how to join in and feels that his asthma is the cause of his social isolation and the curse of his life.

Scott should have been encouraged to develop appropriate and manageble outlets for his activities, using whatever level of tolerance he had. If he had been taught that not all sports activities are equally prone to produce asthma, his story might have been a much different and happier one.

Families with asthmatics require social and emotional support. Physicians could provide this but all too often they attend only to the physical exam and the prescriptions. They may not have the time, the interest, or even the competence to deal with psychosocial situations. We once asked 10 mothers, referred to us because their children had severe chronic asthma, whether their physicians had ever questioned or talked to them about exercise and physical activity for the child. In every instance the reply was the same: "Well, of course the doctor agrees that my child cannot participate in sports." For these mothers the fear of asthma, compounded by medical advice, fostered a needlessly overprotective attitude.

Doctors must bring out into the open and help dispel the crippling attitudes and the negative feelings asthma generates. They must openly and forthrightly discuss the guilt and the fear that frequently accompany asthma in order to counteract the overprotection with which families often smother asthmatic members.

Good and Bad Sports

Activities vary greatly in their ability to induce asthma. Some physicians have always encouraged physical activity, but until recently most doctors have not. This attitude began to change in 1958 when a group, which has come to be called "Bucking Bronchos" (because they advocate bucking bronchial asthma), developed an exercise program for asthmatics that combines gymnastics, basketball, and swimming.

Swimming is the best exercise for asthmatics and among the best of all types of physical conditioners; many with severe asthma are outstanding competitive swimmers. Running is the worst form of exercise for asthma. The reason for the difference is not known, but there are some good clues. For one thing, the higher the temperature the less likely you are to have exercise-induced asthma. Jogging in Boston in December is much more likely to result in wheezing than jogging in Honolulu in December. Humidity also appears to be a factor. The higher the humidity of the outside air, the better off you are. Someone who swims has the advantage of exercising in agreeably warm, humid conditions, while runners breathe outside ambient air, which may be cold and extremely low in humidity.

We strongly endorse swimming and urge parents to introduce their asthmatic children to a regular program in which they can learn to swim and become competent and confident doing it. Learning to swim not only provides good physical conditioning and training but, more important, increases confidence and gives children something in which they can perform competently.

Continuous, sustained effort, even in the mildest form, is more likely to provoke an asthma attack than repeated, interrupted sessions. A brisk one-mile walk to buy a newspaper is more likely to cause wheezing than interrupted jogs of 50 yards; that is — jog 50 yards, rest, then jog 50 more yards. Thus, bursts of activity followed by rest can often be tolerated. Weight training provides this kind of experience; aerobics does not.

Where exercise-induced asthma is aggravated by cold weather, a 3M cold weather mask (available from your pharmacy) or a muffler increases the humidity of inhaled air and reduces the intensity of the symptoms; breathing through the nose also helps.

A PHYSICAL TRAINING PROGRAM FOR ASTHMATICS

We encourage asthmatics to follow a regular daily program of exercise performed at the same time each day. The exercise (swimming, weight training, martial arts, gymnastics) should intersperse periods of activity and rest and should not exceed 30 to 45 minutes. Keep a record of what you do and set goals (i.e., so many laps in the pool by Christmas, so many curls or presses each week). Begin slowly and gradually increase. Remember that short intense periods of exercise are less likely to induce wheezing than prolonged uninterrupted exercise, even if only mild.

Everyone should be allowed to choose their own sport or activity depending on their skills, their schedules, their physical size, and their aspirations. There is almost no sport, except scuba diving, that should be excluded. (We know one proficient asthmatic scuba diver who has had no problems, but we do not recommend it. Scuba diving for asthmatics is potentially lethal.)

For most individuals, the ideal goal is to participate in team sports. If you are the parent of an asthmatic child, try to put aside your concerns and help him or her attend a competition or game even if he or she wheezed a little that morning. The emotional trauma of not participating may be as likely to induce wheezing as the activity itself.

Many team sports are available, even for very small children. All school children participate, not just the gifted few. Regrettably, as children get to junior high school age and beyond, the competition may make participation less enjoyable for many. This is especially true of varsity football and basketball, but there are intramural sports — in particular, soccer, swimming, and tennis — in which all children can participate.

Justin had asthma with intense periods of wheezing from the time he was one year of age. By the time he was three he knew that exercise would make him wheeze. His parents signed him up for soccer while he was in kindergarten. At first he was very enthusiastic, particularly when his parents bought his uniform. However, as the time for the first game approached, he invented all sorts of excuses to avoid going. His father encouraged him just to go and watch, but Justin was embarrassed at the prospect of being seen standing on the sidelines. Finally, about 20 minutes before the first match, Justin's father told him that he could play for the first few minutes of the game and then just tell the coach that he did not feel well. Justin agreed to go but still was reluctant. However, once they got to the game and Justin began playing he forgot all about his fears. He was having too much fun. With a lot of encouragement from his parents, which they patiently provided before each game, Justin finally learned to accept his fear and limitations and to experience the pure enjoyment of participation. Team sports did a tremendous amount for his morale and self-confidence.

Other activities asthmatics can perform include bicycling and hiking. A warm-up beforehand will reduce chances of wheezing and shortness of breath. As a precaution, exercise or competitive sports should be avoided under certain conditions, such as when pollen or air pollution is high or when respiratory infections are present. A wind-down period at the end of the game or activity is also useful in forestalling attacks of wheezing and other breathing difficulties.

Exercise for Severe Asthmatics

A few children have such severe asthma that they are unable to participate in regular competitive or training programs in their community, or the community may not have the resources to condition and help such children out. In these instances physical activity supervised by parents at home — breathing exercises, short periods of training, and learning to swim — may help. Even so, some children who are dependent on steroids and other heavy medications simply cannot participate. In those instances it may be useful to consider special training. Throughout the United States there are a large number of summer camps for asthmatics. They are discussed in Chapter 18. The *Asthma Resources Directory* (see Appendix H) contains a list of these camps.

Regular exercise increases fitness, not just of lungs but the heart too. Adolescents, particularly those who have had severe asthma in childhood, will often have poor muscle development, and the rare child may have chest deformities. Programs of physical activity that include conditioning the upper torso should be started for all these children.

Using Medication in the Prevention or Treatment of Exercise-Induced Asthma

Exercise-induced asthma is no different from any other form of bronchospasm, and the drugs used to control it are the ones described and discussed in Chapter 15. The first step is to determine whether exercise is the only factor or one of a number of factors implicated in wheezing. If exercise is not the only factor, make certain that you or your child is receiving the best drugs available; that may be all that is necessary to prevent or reduce the exercise-induced problems. Verify that you have the correct dose of theophylline or beta agonists and that you are using the beta agonist effectively. Determine whether you need cromolyn or a metered aerosol steroid or even an oral steroid. Your doctor should listen carefully to your chest and do pulmonary function testing at rest to determine if you have some limited reserve and wheezing.

If on the other hand your wheezing is *only* associated with exercise, the problem becomes much simpler. The only issue then is to decide whether to carry and use medication prior to exercise. Theophyllines, beta agonists, and cromolyn all prevent exercise-induced wheezing when taken before exercise. However, there is a complication: children are usually forbidden to carry medication to school and may hesitate or be embarrassed to ask the school nurse for drugs. Help them work out an effective arrangement with school personnel. Remind them that it is less embarrassing to ask to take their medication than to suffer the consequences, either of not taking it or of not participating.

When medication to prevent exercise-induced asthma is indicated, we recommend the following:

1. *Beta agonists,* particularly when given as a metered aerosol (not in pill or capsule form), are the most effective drugs against exercise-induced asthma. We prefer beta agonists because they are easy to take, have no irritant effect, and, with reasonable care, cannot result in overdose.
2. *Cromolyn,* or sodium cromoglycate, because of its lack of systemic effects, is often preferred in the pretreatment of exercise-induced asthma in children and adults. Taking it presents some difficulty, which makes it less useful than the more effectively packaged beta agonists. Nonetheless, when used correctly, it works well in many people.
3. *Theophyllines* provide protection for exercise-induced asthma, but they act slowly and require large doses well in advance of the activity.

Atropine-like drugs (for example, Atrovent) seem *not* to protect against exercise-induced asthma; steroids, when taken prior to exercise, *do not* prevent wheezing or shortness of breath.

The effect of these drugs may be very short term. Whereas this is all that is needed for virtually all children, there are some sports or activities in which longer-term therapy is needed. Obviously, this would require round-the-clock protection prior to participation. The use of cromolyn, or else the long-acting theophyllines, in appropriate doses, is recommended in these instances.

CHAPTER

10 Surgery, Anesthesia, and Asthma

Asthmatics, like all other individuals before surgery, must have an intensive preoperative evaluation to make sure that their bodies can withstand the trauma involved. Because surgery often involves assisted ventilation and reduced respiratory capacity, the asthmatic may be particularly at risk. In addition, because asthmatics may be on medications, some alternative method must be found for any period of time in which they are not allowed to take anything by mouth.

PRE-SURGICAL EVALUATION

There are a number of factors to take into account in the pre-surgery evaluation. Although emotion does not cause asthma, emotional responses that cause hyperventilation may make asthma worse. The apprehension experienced in the days prior to entering the hospital and in the hours immediately before the operation may trigger an asthmatic response and intense bronchospasm. It is important, therefore, that you fully under-stand the nature of the surgery or procedure being done and the reasons for it. Knowing exactly what is to be faced dispels fear and insecurity. If you are afraid, if you do not understand, if you need additional counsel, let your doctor know.

With careful planning, some of the risks for asthmatics associated with surgery can be anticipated and held to a minimum. Some anesthetic agents are capable of provoking an asthmatic attack either during the induction phase (when you are first being put to sleep) or during the actual period of use of anesthetic agents. For this reason, anticipating and skirting this potential hazard is vital. During the induction phase your physician may choose to use diazepam or ketamine — relaxants which reduce pre-operative stress. Or he or she may administer inhalation treatment with the anesthetic halothane. Short-acting barbiturate-like drugs like thiopental ought to be avoided because they may produce a cough and bronchospasm. *It is up to you to routinely advise all doctors that you have asthma, even if it is very mild.* Also make sure that everyone concerned knows what drugs you routinely take. Do not assume that you can use them freely in the hospitals, though. Hospitals confiscate medications and permit them to be administered only by staff.

ANESTHETICS

In pulmonary anesthesia, the most common form, the only agents that are routinely ruled out for asthmatics are cyclopropane and nitrous oxide. Cyclopropane is not used because it can produce irregularities in the heartbeat, which may be intensified in individuals taking beta agonists or theophylline for their asthma. Nitrous oxide, or laughing gas, a drug used for many years as an anesthetic agent, is avoided because it makes asthma worse. Other anesthetics routinely used such as halothane and enflurane apparently do not produce an increase in wheezing during surgery. Halothane may produce some dilation of airways, which could actually help asthma.

Anesthesia can also be produced by injection or intravenous introduction of drugs that directly block nerves. Virtually all of the neuromuscular blocking agents, curare and succinyl choline among them, release histamine. In patients with asthma, this could represent a serious complication as histamine release may cause bronchospasm, although it occurs only rarely in surgery. As long as your surgeon and anesthesiologist know about your asthma and prior bad reactions you have had to medications, the odds are overwhelming that you will be safe. Even if you were to have a reaction, plans for an emergency can be worked out in advance.

Local anesthetics also come into the picture, especially for minor surgery treated on an outpatient basis. Dentists frequently employ locals, especially drugs in the Novocain and lidocaine family. Such drugs may provoke significant allergic reactions including everything from anaphylaxis (acute and intense collapse of the airways) to hives. There is no way of knowing in advance who will have such a reaction, but if you have shown *any* sensitivity to a local anesthetic in the past, discuss it with your physician or dentist and have tests before surgery to determine if in fact you are allergic to the anesthetic slated for use. If so, alternatives can be found.

The most serious problems involve patients who have accidents, are rendered unconscious, and must undergo emergency surgery. If you are in this condition there is nothing you can do or say in your own behalf. If you are an asthmatic and on medication, we urge you to wear a Medic-Alert bracelet so that medical workers will know of your medical problems.*

Harry is a lifelong asthmatic. He controls his symptoms efficiently with intermittent medication. He is also intensely allergic to penicillin and had a serious generalized reaction to it several years ago. At the time his doctor advised Harry to get a Medic-Alert bracelet, but Harry didn't follow through, believing it wasn't worth the trouble and expense. Besides, he didn't want to wear a bracelet.

Five months ago Harry was in an auto accident that put him through the windshield and knocked him unconscious. He was rushed to the hospital with a variety of fractures, cuts, and contusions, and, to avoid infection, the attending doctor began him on antibiotics, including penicillin. Within minutes Harry's respiration became labored and hives blossomed all over his body. The nurse saw the symptoms and alertly stopped the medication and called the doctor. Epinephrine (Adrenalin) was administered and got the symptoms under control in 15 minutes. However, during that quarter hour Harry turned cyanotic (blue) from lack of oxygen and has remained in a coma ever since. It is unclear whether the coma is entirely due to the automobile accident or is the result of severe oxygen deprivation suffered during the adverse reaction to penicillin.

If you have serious allergies, carry warning identification. It may save your life!

The Interactions of Anesthetics and Surgical Drugs with Asthma Medications

The choice of anesthetic agents, as well as of any other medications during surgery, should take into account their potential interactions with asthma drugs. A drug interaction means that drug A, when taken by an individual who is already receiving drug B, may have a different or a more severe effect than usual. Asthmatics on high doses of theophylline, who also use high-dose beta agonists — both asthma medications — may experience irregularities of the heartbeat. An irregular heartbeat may also occur when theophylline is taken along with anesthetic agents.

It is extremely important that you inform your surgeon about *all* drugs you have taken or are taking. Do not omit any. Some have long survival times and may remain present in the body for days. You must also mention illegal or abusive drugs you have used. The doctor needs to know this; such information is kept confidential.

---

* Applications for Medic-Alert bracelets are available in physicians' offices or hospitals, or they may be secured from the Medic-Alert Foundation, P.O. Box 1009, Turlock, CA 95381.

OTHER DANGERS IN SURGERY

An operation produces a significant amount of stress for the body. It can — and often does — interfere with normal eating and drinking patterns. During recovery, when you cannot take anti-asthma drugs by mouth it may be important to continue these drugs. Eliminating steroids, for instance, may result in a catastrophic return of asthma symptoms. In addition, if people who take steroids are stressed during surgery they may no longer have the capacity to produce cortisone of their own to meet the surgically produced challenge. If they cannot respond to the surgical trauma, their blood pressure may fall and they may develop abnormalities in the electrolytic balance of their body fluids. They may even suffer secondary failure of organs including the kidney. Accordingly, it is not uncommon for physicians to provide asthmatics who are on steroids with extra amounts of it, often intravenously, immediately prior to surgery. They may continue steroids in this form for a few days after surgery. *This is important standard practice and is meant to protect you.*

> Tim has never liked to take cortisone, fearing its side effects. He has always preferred a slight wheeze in lieu of taking this drug. Several years ago when inhaled metered-dose cortisone-like drugs appeared, he was elated. For the first time he could have many of the benefits of cortisone with virtually none of its side effects. Thus it was with considerable consternation that Tim found out his doctor was giving him high-dose intravenous steroids immediately before his disc operation. He flatly refused to take the steroids. The nurse tried to contact the doctor, who was not available. The steroids were not given and the surgery had to be postponed. When the doctor heard about this, he explained the need for the short-term steroids to Tim, who finally agreed to their use. Tim should have found out before surgery what to expect, but his doctor should also have explained beforehand and was negligent in not doing so.

Patients with asthma may also have some compromise of their lungs. This may be a result of long-standing asthma or of asthmatic or bronchospastic problems immediately prior to surgery. You should take as much respiratory reserve as possible into the operating room. This means that your asthma therapy should be optimized in the weeks, days, and hours prior to your operation. Your surgeon should test your respiratory reserve well in advance of surgery. For those patients who have chronic problems with mucus production and secretions, it is a good idea in the weeks before surgery to follow faithfully the exercises we describe in Chapter 14 in order to make it easier for you to eliminate the troublesome mucus. If you are likely to have respiratory therapy after surgery, find out beforehand what will be done and exactly how it will be carried out. Ask what being on a respirator will be like, how it will feel, and what you can do to make yourself more comfortable. If necessary insist on trying it out *before* the surgery takes place.

11 Pregnancy and Asthma

Pregnant women with moderate to severe chronic asthma often experience serious qualms about the adverse effects their disease and its treatment may have on them or their child. Yet, by observing a few precautions, there is no reason to avoid or fear pregnancy. In principle, the pregnant asthmatic should be aware of and observe the same cautions any other asthmatic would who was about to undergo medical or surgical procedure (see preceding chapter).

It is of paramount importance that your body be ready for the strain of giving birth. Be prepared both emotionally and physically for the event and be sure your asthma is managed as adequately as possible. Your respiratory reserves should be brought up to the best level available, and you should work to improve your breathing in order to reduce secretions and increase your lung responses and airway capacity. Inform your obstetrician that you have asthma and what, if anything, you are doing for it. In addition, keep the physician who looks after your asthma informed about your pregnancy and the medications you are taking.

USING ASTHMA MEDICATIONS DURING PREGNANCY

It is important both to you and to your baby that you know all you can about the drugs you are taking. Unhappily, despite the millions of women who have asthma, only a handful of scientific studies have assessed the effects on the fetus of drugs used to control asthma during pregnancy. The side effects of many new drugs are only evaluated in men, because experimenters wish to avoid potential abnormalities in the fetus; similarly, drug manufacturers don't want to run the risk of a woman becoming pregnant during drug trials. This precaution is understandable, but it puts asthmatic mothers and their physicians in a dilemma. Although physicians want to treat their asthmatic patients the best way they can, they also want to avoid possible ill effects on the developing baby, and they do not have the information they need to make informed and risk-free decisions. Fortunately, a fair amount of data are available from animal studies, but just because a drug appears safe in pregnant animals does not mean it is safe for humans. Because drug testing is so expensive, all newer drugs for the treatment of asthma come with the warning that they have *not* been tested on pregnant women, and their effect on the fetus is therefore unknown.

Some drugs often prescribed for women with asthma may affect the fetus. Those who have asthma along with recurrent respiratory infections are often treated with the antibiotic tetracycline. This antibiotic *should not* be used during pregnancy because it may affect the teeth and the bones of the baby. Any drugs or compounds that contain too much iodine should also be discontinued, because iodine can affect the development of the thyroid gland in the baby. If too much iodine is taken (iodine is often found in cough syrups), it may even induce a goiter in the mother. Her baby could be born with severely reduced thyroid function which, if undetected and untreated, could cause cretinism.

Several other drugs used in allergies have also been shown to be harmful to the fetus. They include the decongestant phenylephrine and the antihistamines phenylpropanolamine and brompheniramine. These latter three drugs may be found in over-the-counter medications. Therefore, be very careful if you are pregnant or even if you think you might be pregnant.

Beta agonists, theophyllines, cromolyn, and steroids are routinely used in treating chronic asthma. Theophyllines, which are very similar to caffeine, have been used for many years and have been taken by thousands if not millions of pregnant women. Although not studied rigorously, theophylline has *not* been associated with fetal abnormalities. However, beta agonists, including ephedrine, metaproternol, and terbutaline, have not been approved for use during pregnancy because they have not been studied. Cromolyn, which is comparatively safe and free of side effects, has not been studied during pregnancy either. Oral steroids do have the potential for exerting harmful effects on the fetus, particularly if taken in the first trimester of pregnancy. Topical steroids are safer but have not been studied during pregnancy.

We do not wish to alarm pregnant asthmatic women unnecessarily. Because some drugs have not been studied does not mean they are harmful. Allergists and chest physicians often find it necessary to treat pregnant patients with these drugs and have not reported any obvious developmental defects in the babies. Limited studies in animals suggest that these drugs are probably safe. Nevertheless, try to determine the lowest amount of medication needed to effectively relieve your asthma. We would much prefer to treat a pregnant woman whose asthma is well controlled by drugs

102

AVOIDING ASTHMA'S
COMMON AND
UNCOMMON CAUSES
AND
COMPLICATIONS

than a woman who is not on medication but whose asthma is poorly controlled. The latter is much more likely to experience problems — including asthmatic ones — during delivery. Delivery complications (bleeding, infection, prolonged labor due to blood oxygen insufficiency which reduces the muscle tone of the uterus) more than any other single birth experience are likely to exert harmful effects on the baby.

The most dangerous drugs for the fetus are illicit recreational drugs such as cocaine and heroin. "Crack babies," as they are called, are premature, small, addicted, and more likely to die. These drugs should never be used.

Some women elect to have a therapeutic abortion, which is sometimes carried out with drugs that contain prostaglandin-like materials. These prostaglandins can induce severe bronchospasm and *should be avoided* in anybody with asthma.

Because asthma affects from 5 to 13 pregnant women per 1000, most obstetricians know how to deal with asthma during pregnancy. And, interestingly, a pregnant woman experiences some natural improvement in the anatomy of her respiratory system during pregnancy. In addition, the fetus manufactures a special form of hemoglobin that makes fetal red blood cells highly efficient in receiving oxygen from the mother. If the mother has chronic asthma during pregnancy, she may not have enough oxygen; her asthma problem may be aggravated because the fetus, through its special hemoglobin, protects itself at the expense of the mother. Even in women who have moderate to severe chronic asthma during pregnancy, the fetus usually receives enough oxygen.

This subject of oxygen delivered to the fetus may have special relevance to some women. Stress to your oxygen delivery capabilities — such as too vigorous exercise, climbing to extremely high altitudes, or flying in an aircraft without oxygen — may starve you of oxygen and therefore dangerously reduce the baby's oxygen supply. You, the expectant mother, should also have adequate hemoglobin, so that oxygen can be delivered effectively. During the first evaluation for pregnancy, have a complete blood count. If you are found to be anemic, it is important that the reason for the anemia be found out and corrected. Most often it is an iron deficiency. Because a number of nutritional demands are placed on women during pregnancy, it is important for you and your baby that you take multivitamins with iron.

Joann has been happily married for 16 years and has four healthy children. No one would suspect that she suffers from asthma. Her purse is filled with metered aerosols, cromolyn spinhalers, and theophyllines. She wears a Medic-Alert bracelet so that in an emergency doctors will know what drugs she takes, and she strictly avoids the causes of her asthma. At the onset of her first pregnancy her obstetrician told her that as an asthmatic she could forget about natural childbirth. When she asked for reasons her obstetrician was cryptic and abrupt and did not answer her question. He put her off with an admonition not to worry. Joann called her allergist, who recommended another obstetrician who had no qualms about natural childbirth in asthmatics. Joann's active participation in her own health care is an important part of her successful coping with asthma.

ALLERGY SHOTS AND PREGNANCY

As we point out in Chapter 16, the use of allergy shots for the treatment of asthma is controversial. It is clear that allergy shots may relieve allergic rhinitis (hay fever). However, the twitchiness of airways is not always improved by allergy shots.

Allergy shots may also cause an acute allergic reaction, or anaphylaxis. These episodes can be extraordinarily harmful, even fatal, to a pregnant woman and may induce spontaneous abortion. For this reason allergy shots should *not* be started during pregnancy. Moreover, if you are already receiving allergy shots, do *not* increase the dose. Maintain the same safe level you were receiving at the time your pregnancy was confirmed. That way you reap the benefits of the shots without running the risks attendant to increased concentrations and the possibly acute reactions to them.

AFTER THE BABY COMES

Many experts today agree that breast-feeding, if possible, is most beneficial to mother and child. Breast-fed babies show better rates of development and a lower incidence of infection and allergies than those who are placed on formula early. With lactating asthmatic mothers, however, some of the drugs taken to combat the asthma may cross over to the infant and cause undesirable side effects. What drugs to take and the dosage should be worked out carefully with the pediatrician or family practitioner. Some of the drugs likely to be taken by asthmatic mothers and the possible effects on their breast-fed children are listed in Table 10 on the following page.

TABLE 10 Drugs and Breast-Feeding

Drug	Possible Effects on Breast-Fed Child
Alcohol (beer is often recommended to help in production of milk; alcohol appears as a vehicle in many OTC medications)	Atypical development, drowsiness, deep sleep, weakness
Ephedrine (in decongestants and some beta agonists)	Irritability, excessive crying, disturbed sleep
Caffeine (in coffee, tea, cola, OTC cold medications)	Irritability, poor sleep patterns
Theophylline	Irritability, poor sleep patterns; rarely, vomiting, seizure, hemorrhaging
Theobromine (in coffee, tea, cocoa or chocolate)	Said to cause irritability, colic; interacts with theophylline and heightens its side effects
Salicylates (aspirin)	Respiratory distress, very rapid breathing, restlessness
Iodine (may come from radioactive studies, cough medicines, decongestants)	Drowsiness, lethargy, goiter
Prednisone, other steroids	Lowered adrenal function
Heroin, cocaine, marijuana, methamphetamines	Retarded growth, addiction

CARING
FOR YOUR
ASTHMA

Self-Help for People with Asthma

WHAT IS SELF-MANAGEMENT?

Self-management* is not a new idea. Every asthma sufferer decides (or has someone else decide) how to manage his or her complaint. Whereas some individual attempts at self-management of moderate to severe asthma have proved satisfactory, more often they have not worked as well as they might. Recent work has turned up a number of useful principles and self-care procedures that apply particularly well to asthma sufferers. These new findings, when put into practice, are much more likely to result in successful self-help and all of its side benefits — effective, timely, and economical treatment; fewer emergency room visits; better school or job attendance; less disability; and shorter bouts of illness.

To become competent in self-management you need to work faithfully and intelligently at what sometimes may seem to be repetitive, unnecessary tasks. After such training, effective decisions about care of asthma can be made by children as young as six, providing their parents are coached in ways of offering support. You will have to make difficult and occasionally frightening choices; yet, if conscientious about it, you have every reason to expect to gain more control of your life, to feel better physically and better about yourself, to live more fully, and to cut your medical costs significantly.

The competencies you need to establish in order to take charge of your asthma are

---

*We use the words self-management, self-care, and self-help interchangeably, to mean a process wherein you act as your own primary health provider, taking the steps necessary to prevent, detect, and treat illness.

- *Accepting responsibility* for managing your own self
- *Acquiring the information* that permits you to prevent, detect, and treat your illness
- *Perfecting your decision-making skills* so that you know what to do about your asthma and when to do it, and have confidence in your ability to do it
- *Developing awareness* of your bodily processes and how to control them
- *Building a support network* of family, peers, and professionals

Accepting Responsibility for Self-Care

Sharing health care decisions or placing the whole burden for them on others (including one's doctor) is commonplace. By doing this we avoid responsibility for acts and decisions while freeing ourselves to blame others when things go wrong. Taking responsibility for your asthma (and getting rid of the temptation to cast blame) is the single most difficult yet liberating step on the road to self-management of your asthma. Once you are ready to accept the fact that you have an illness and therefore can make decisions and choices about its treatment and course, mastering the other competencies is relatively easy.

There are a number of fundamental points that you must understand fully and accept without reservation. First, you and you alone have the *right* to make decisions about your own health care; what form it will take, when and by whom it will be administered. After all, you, more than anyone else, are the one most directly and profoundly affected by these decisions.

Second, you alone have the final *responsibility* for making health care decisions affecting you. Allowing someone else (including your doctor) to exercise that responsibility is unfair to the other person and severely limits your own freedom, autonomy, and sense of self-worth and self-control.

Third, you have or can acquire the *competence* to make wise, informed decisions about your own health care. You know your own symptoms and your history and are in a better position than anyone else to judge the likely consequences of decisions, whatever they may be.

Finally, with training and practice you can develop the *confidence* and *willingness* to accept the consequences — favorable and unfavorable — of decisions you make in your own behalf. Take comfort from the fact that most of your decisions will be the right ones, and if you do slip up you can profit from the learning opportunity it provides.

The decision chart depicted in Figure 7 will help you to establish your readiness to accept and claim responsibility for your own self-care and to assert your own independence.

Sometimes discussions with doctors or parents or other individuals who are making treatment decisions for you do not turn out as you had hoped

FIGURE 7 Steps to Independence

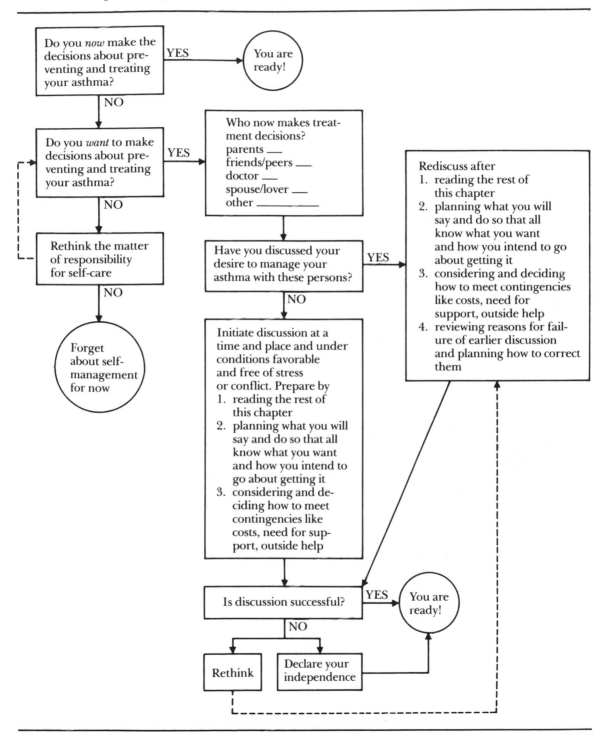

they would. Therefore, it is often useful to go back and try to find the reasons for your failure to communicate. The most common ones are

- Not explaining your needs, rights, and wishes clearly and persuasively
- Not having the argument or point of view you put forward accepted, considered, or even heard by the other party
- Not having effective replies to arguments or points brought out by the other party

Careful preparation and planning can help you to anticipate and overcome these problems. Strategies to follow, depending on the consequences of actions, are suggested in Figure 7. In addition, it helps to bear in mind the usefulness of tactics that can maintain the discussion. If you meet with resistance, calmly ask for a fuller explanation of the reasons for it. To comprehend or clarify the other person's opposition, use statements like "As I get it, you don't want me to do this because. . . . Is that a fair way of putting it?" Work to understand (and have the other person understand) your wishes and needs clearly, fairly, and dispassionately. Steer away from haggling or quarreling over small points that simply sidetrack or polarize the discussion.

Acquiring Information to Detect, Prevent, and Treat Asthma

Detection

You are the best source of information about your asthma. Often you can determine the cause of your symptoms simply by being observant about yourself and your reactions. Once that cause is identified you are well on your way to adequate prevention and treatment. Chapter 5 details procedures for you to follow in order to pinpoint the cause of your asthma.

Finding the Right Doctor

If you do not succeed on your own in locating the cause of your allergy, it is time to consider getting an allergist to help you. Your family doctor who can recommend someone should be consulted first. Chapter 13 tells you what to look for in selecting a doctor. Choose your doctor carefully, because he or she will be an important member of the support network we discuss later on in this chapter. You will want to find someone who will help you and trust you to manage your own symptoms. Not every allergist is willing to allow you this kind of freedom and support. Before anything else is settled, tell the allergist exactly what you want. If he or she is unwilling to cooperate with your wishes, find someone else who will. (Medical school departments of allergy or allergy departments of teaching hospitals will know the names of doctors who are interested in promoting patient self-management.) Remember that it is your *right* to be responsible for your own health care decisions.

Prevention

Avoiding the offending agent is the key to preventing the onset of asthma attacks. Chapter 6 specifies steps you can take to avoid, or at least cut down the risk of coming into contact with, the substances that provoke your reaction. Unfortunately, for a few problems (pollen-caused asthma, for example), it may be impossible. For most, however, avoidance is possible but may be inconvenient and perhaps a nuisance. You will have to assert yourself — ask what is in or on foods, decline to eat particular dishes, ask that windows be kept shut, request that people not smoke, and so on. In circumstances where others are not prepared to make these concessions you must be ready to remove yourself from the endangering environment — avoid means *avoid*, and for an asthma sufferer, nothing else suffices.

Taking sensible precautions makes this difficult process easier. Going on a picnic during pollen season (no matter how much you would enjoy it) simply invites illness, unless your asthma is under good medical control. If you have exercise-induced asthma, participating in a sport or game you know will soon have you wheezing is obviously unwise. However, intelligent use of medication before exercise can often enable you to participate without discomfort. At certain times of the year you may need to wear a conspicuous dust and pollen mask. If in addition to catching pollens it also catches the attention of a lot of gawking people, wear it anyway. It's better to be conspicuous than sick. Respecting and accommodating your illness (and asking others to do the same) makes it more possible for you to live a normal and satisfying life.

Treatment

Treatment refers to actions you take, or help another to take, to control or get rid of your asthmatic symptoms. Such actions include regular exercise, breathing training, medication, stress-reducing activities, and the like. For the sake of your safety and well-being, adopt these measures only after you receive medical advice. This is especially true if your condition is chronic, moderate to severe, and, as with so many asthmatic complaints, potentially life-threatening.

The problem with treatment is not so much *knowing* what to do as *doing* it. An astonishing number of people neglect to stick to treatment schedules, fail to follow directions, stop taking treatment before they should, or give up on treatment because of troublesome but minor side effects or because they want to test to see whether they are "cured." Figure 8 spells out some of the major questions or problems associated with nonadherence to treatment procedures and indicates what steps you can take to support and reinforce your commitment to maintain your treatment program.

FIGURE 8 Adhering to Treatment Procedures

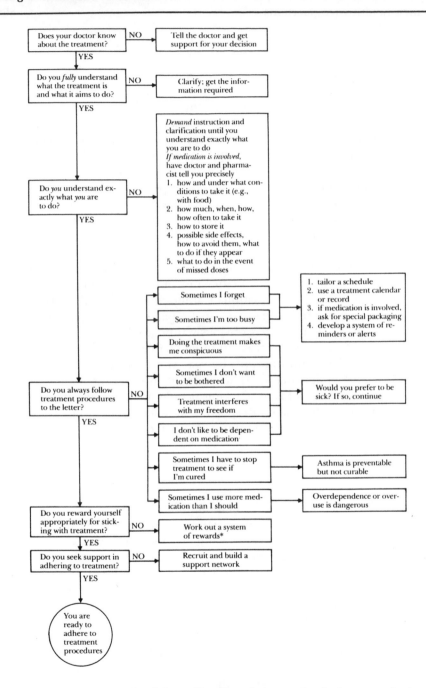

*Rewards can include relaxation or recreational time off, saving tokens or coins for later use, sharing knowledge of compliance with a supportive relative or friend, self-praise, small treats, etc.

PERFECTING YOUR DECISION-MAKING SKILLS

Making decisions is an important element in self-care. Although you may want to have more input about decisions that affect you, your illness, and your life-style, you may be unaccustomed to doing so. Thus, the prospect of decision-making may seem unsafe or overwhelming. Figure 9 presents a sound set of guidelines for you to follow in order to make sensible decisions.

Most of the time defining the problem (the first step in the process) presents no difficulties. You will be faced with a straightforward question like "What must I do successfully to treat (or avoid or control) my asthmatic symptoms?" There are definitely positive, constructive things you can do. However, there will be occasions when the problems are less clear-cut and more troublesome. This often happens when an element of conflict is

FIGURE 9 Improving Decision-Making

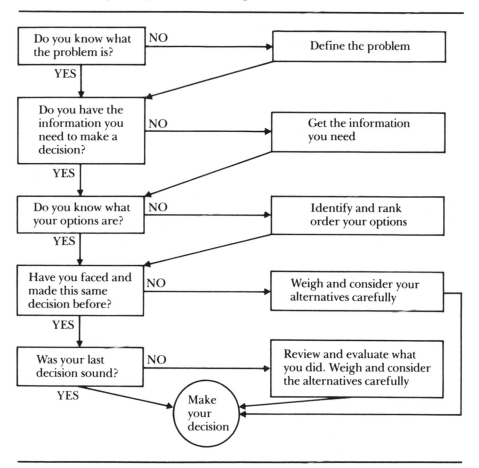

involved, when any action you might take has both positive and negative aspects. For example, there is the recurrent question about whether or not to keep taking a medication. Most people simply do not like to be dependent on medication. If you are controlling your symptoms through regular use of a drug, and if a period of time goes by during which you are free of symptoms, you may be strongly tempted to reduce or cut out the medication entirely, either in the belief that you are "cured" or just to see if you can get along without it.

When this sort of situation crops up it should be clear to you what the problem is — what exactly are you trying to achieve, prevent, or prove? Once having formulated it ("Can I get along without medication?"), you can then move on to the next step, which is to consider how to arrive at an answer. One way, of course, is just to stop and see what happens. Perhaps nothing will happen, or nothing right away, or you will relapse, possibly seriously. A better, safer tactic to follow entails first finding out what others (especially your allergist) think of the possibility and what has happened to you (or others like you) who tried to stop medication in the past. If the results are unhappy, clearly the odds favor continuing the medication, even though it is tiresome and appears to be unnecessary.

With the problem clarified, the information you need can be found fairly easily. Read widely about asthma and medications, ask your doctor, compare your experience with fellow sufferers. The National Jewish Center for Immunology and Respiratory Medicine (see Appendix G) in Denver, Colorado, has established Lung Line, a telephone information service that dispenses information on respiratory disease to callers. By dialing their toll-free number, 1-800-222-LUNG, you can find out about developments in asthma treatment including new medications, recent research findings, and facts on other questions related to the Center's specialties. This individualized, responsive, sympathetic service has been enthusiastically endorsed by its users. Most important, do not forget to trust and to take into account what you already know about yourself and your complaint.

In getting information together develop a clear idea of the options available to you and the consequences, negative and positive, attached to each one. Also, think back and see if you have had to face this problem before and how you handled it. If what you did worked, fine; if not, you will want to go with one of the alternatives.

The decision-making process calls on you to think clearly and carefully and to take action that grows out of knowledge, analysis, and experience. If you do this you will be rewarded with sound, effective choices.

DEVELOPING AWARENESS OF AND CONTROL OVER BODILY PROCESSES

There are dozens of processes going on inside the body all the time, and we are quite oblivious to most of them. It is possible to become more conscious of them, however, and to use this knowledge to manage your asthmatic reactions more effectively. In particular, it will be useful for you to learn the signs — the small changes in the way you feel or react — that precede an asthmatic attack. You may already be aware of these faint premonitory changes. If you are not, learning what they are will give you the chance to take preventive steps before you are into a full-blown reaction.

The ASTHMA EARLY WARNING INDICATOR (Figure 10) will help you to pick out the signals or triggers of an impending asthmatic reaction if you do not already know them. To complete it, go back over your most recent episode. Try very hard to remember the sensations or other bodily signs that *preceded* the full onset of your symptoms. In the appropriate spaces check all the prodromal symptoms you can recall. Then keep the same record for the next three episodes. After the record is completed, examine it carefully; note any recurring patterns and monitor them every day. Once you can read your bodily signs with enough accuracy to forecast impending reactions, you can prevent or control them. Learn how to use a PEF meter (see Chapter 5).

By now all this record-keeping (to identify, anticipate, and ward off your symptoms) may make it seem like most of your time will be spent filling out forms. Like most kinds of detection, success in identifying and steering clear of whatever is producing asthmatic reactions depends pretty much on being methodical, trying not to overlook anything, and analyzing critically and open-mindedly all the information you collect. The forms we supply take very little time to maintain: a few minutes at the end of each day. But the payoff can be extravagantly beneficial.

Behavioral Control

Many of the symptoms that accompany asthma — the breathing difficulties, for instance — can be greatly improved through behavioral control of bodily processes.

Behavioral control is nothing more than a training process that enables you to exert more voluntary control over certain bodily activities. A number of simple breathing exercises, for example, materially help to counteract the bronchospasms brought on by emotion and hyperventilation in asthma; a variety of relaxation techniques blunt the fear reactions that accompany and intensify asthmatic attacks. The dread of injections (which often provokes or heightens allergic shot reactions) can also be mastered by practicing these easily learned skills.

Biofeedback — a process in which you are able to monitor and observe the effect of conscious efforts to regulate air flow, blood pressure, pulse, and level of stress or tension — is a technologically somewhat more advanced method of achieving behavioral control of asthmatic symptoms.

If it is apparent that some form of behavioral control will help you take charge of your asthma, your physician may be able to refer you to appro-

FIGURE 10   ASTHMA EARLY WARNING INDICATOR

Check (✓) any sign that preceded each of the last four episodes; double check (✓✓) any that occurred 24 hours or less before the episode.

Type of Reaction	Specific Signs or Indicators	Noticed during Episode:				No. of ✓s	Comments or Hunches
		1	2	3	4		
Pulmonary	PEF readings in red or yellow*						Episode 1:
	Tightness in chest						
	Shortness of breath						
	Wheezing						
	Cough						
	Mucus in chest						Episode 2:
Ear, Nose, and Throat	Runny nose						
	Nasal congestion						
	Earache/inflammation						
	Scratchy or sore throat						Episode 3:
Psychological	Irritable						
	Hyperactive/excitable						
	Anxious/depressed						
Other	Headache						Episode 4:
	Tiredness/fatigue						
	Muscle pain/cramps						
	Low-grade fever						
	Restless sleep						

*For instructions on using a peak expiratory flow (PEF) meter see page 43.

priate resources. If not, your local college or university counseling center will know of psychologists in the community who are familiar with and use behavioral techniques.

BUILDING A SUPPORT NETWORK OF FAMILY, PEERS, AND PROFESSIONALS

You who suffer from asthma will be immensely aided in your efforts toward self-management if you recruit a support network of family, friends, fellow sufferers, and professionals who understand your problem, trust your ability to look after yourself, and stand ready to help you if and when the need arises. Such whole-hearted, unconditional support of family members and others important to you, along with your own belief that what you are doing will have beneficial results, is absolutely essential to the success of your efforts.

Family and friends often fail to be adequately supportive because they do not understand your complaint and your needs. They may reject your asthma or resent it because of the burden of cost or inconvenience that it imposes. They may tell you that you are malingering or that your symptoms are either imaginary or the result of some emotional or psychological shortcoming that you could get over if you but tried. They may even go so far as to blame themselves for your illness. They may harbor doubts or reservations about the effectiveness of the prevention or treatment procedures you are following. This attitude is easily detected, and sensing it may cause you to lose faith in what you are doing. This in turn may encourage you to be careless or lackadaisical about adhering to the procedures you *must* observe strictly if you are to take charge of your allergies.

These serious misunderstandings can only be overcome by straightforward communication. Explain how you feel, what it is you want and need from them, and what they should expect in return. For instance, asthma produces thick mucus which blocks airways. This blockage is serious and asthmatics struggle to get the mucus up in an attempt to clear the airways. To others, this struggle can be offensive. Parents or friends who feel this way may openly criticize you or try to prevent you from producing mucus, not realizing that this (to them) disgusting activity is immensely helpful to you, the asthmatic. They need to be made aware of this and helped to put aside their disapproving attitude in favor of one that will tolerate or even encourage or aid it. Explaining the facts should be enough; but you, on your part, can try and make it easy for others by doing the coughing, hawking, and spitting out of earshot if possible. Your physician may ultimately be your best source of help. He or she can explain what the problem is, how it affects you, and what family and friends can do to be supportive.

If you can find them, among the most useful members of a support network are individuals who have the same problem you do. Increasingly, interest/support groups of asthmatics are being formed. Some of these groups are established by outpatient clinics or hospital allergy departments. They bring together professionals, individuals suffering from the same or closely similar complaints, and (often) their parents. They usually meet periodically to discuss and exchange experiences, share feelings and strategies for coping, and act as backup for one another (via telephone) in the event of problems, questions, or trouble. The freedom to consult, the common experience, and the knowledge that there are others similarly troubled have been shown to be important adjuncts to successful self-management of asthmatic symptoms.

Finally, there are health professionals other than physicians who can be immensely helpful in enabling you to manage your allergy. Psychologists, especially those who specialize in behavioral therapy, provide training and successful experience in relief of a wide range of symptoms; health personnel in school (nurses, psychologists, sports medics) or at work (occupational health or safety personnel, nurses) can help you isolate the causes and make you better able to cope with your complaint.

Medical Care

WHAT TO EXPECT
AT THE DOCTOR'S OFFICE

A complete medical history and an adequate physical examination are vital to the diagnosis and effective management of your or your child's asthma. To get a proper basis for treatment — and possibly to find out what is causing your asthma — your doctor should do three main things: take a careful history, conduct a thorough physical examination, and order some laboratory tests, including an X ray.

> Frances, 67, suddenly develops a persistent cough, pains in the right side of her chest, and a wheeze. Because of the wheezing she is convinced she has asthma. She goes to the drugstore and buys Primatene Mist. After using it for 10 days with no success she decides to see a doctor. By that time Frances is very short of breath. Her doctor listens to her chest and, because he does not hear air movement, orders an X ray. The X ray shows a collapse of part of her right lung. A bronchoscopy is done. During the procedure the doctor extricates a cherry pit that was apparently taken into the lung some time before. Frances does not recollect the event. "I hardly ever eat cherries," she says. "I don't even *like* them."

The Medical History

The medical history is the most important element in the process of finding out whether or not you have asthma and, if you do, what causes it. A good, thorough, well-taken history can and often does establish the validity of the diagnosis of asthma and its causes. You should be prepared to answer the doctor's questions accurately, fully, and honestly. You can anticipate what most of the questions will be by studying the ASTHMA FINDER (Figure 5) in Chapter 5. (This is also a good way to check on how thorough and careful the doctor is in trying to help you. Where important areas are neglected — if your family background goes unchecked, for instance, or if you are not asked about changes in your environment that occurred about the time of your first attack — you should take note.) The doctor will be especially interested in the nature of the onset of your asthma. Was it sudden and unexpected or slow, gradual, and progressive? Was it associated with a fever or infection? Did it show up when you moved or changed your environment at work, home, or school? Do you have any pets? Any new pets? Does your asthma get worse at particular times of the year? Do you smoke? Do some foods seem to trigger your asthma or make it worse? What are they?

The Physical Examination

Your physician should give you a *complete* physical examination. You can get some idea of the caliber of your doctor by taking note of how careful and thorough the physical is. A good doctor (or staff) will carry out the routine steps, such as recording weight, height, pulse, and blood pressure. If you are over 40 the doctor should do a rectal examination; women should have their breasts examined.

Then come the steps that tie in more closely to asthma, beginning with carefully listening to your chest with a stethoscope. (Many physicians believe that, for asthmatics, the stethoscope — and what lies between its ear pieces — is the most powerful diagnostic tool!) If the doctor doesn't listen to your lungs at all or does it in a perfunctory way, you've been short-changed. The lungs are vital to maintaining all systems in your body, and asthma starves the lungs by cutting off the air flow. Thus, asthma can affect the heart, the kidneys, and the skin. Your physician, by combining direct inspection and laboratory testing of these organs and sites, can determine if they have been affected — by chronic lack of oxygen, for example.

Next, an X ray should be taken. This will reveal what your lungs look like and will show up any damage or the presence of other conditions — emphysema, for example — which may be mistaken for asthma. Unfortunately, there are many people who dread and balk at the idea of having a chest X ray, fearing the possibility of cancer. It is true that exposure to a radioactive source can be dangerous and harmful. However, the amount of exposure nowadays is much smaller than it was even a few years ago when the equipment was less sensitive and efficient. The small risk that radiation carries has to be weighed against the real dangers that respiratory problems carry. Tragic errors have occurred because of refusals to have a needed X ray.

Anthony had had asthma all his life and was used to wheezing, which he controlled adequately by taking over-the-counter medications. His doctor frequently advised him that there were much better drugs available, but Anthony paid no attention. He did not like the thought of taking prescription drugs, believing that the over-the-counter remedies were less harmful to him — a surprisingly common error. Even so, at age 40 he was able to live fairly comfortably with his complaint. Then, one afternoon at work, he began to experience aches and chills. He went home, thinking he had the flu. His wife took his temperature, which registered 101.5°. He also noticed that his wheezing was getting worse. That didn't surprise him because it almost always got worse when he had a virus. Next morning his temperature was 102°.

Anthony went to his doctor, who listened to his chest and concluded that Anthony might have pneumonia. He told Anthony he ought to have an X ray and be placed on antibiotics. Anthony refused. The doctor tried to insist and became angry when Anthony refused to comply. Anthony, too, lost his temper and stormed out. That night his fever suddenly shot up to 104° and he became confused and disoriented. His wife called an ambulance and Anthony was taken to the emergency room where an X ray was finally taken. The picture showed severe diffuse bacterial pneumonia. Anthony was admitted to the hospital and started on antibiotics, but not soon enough. He died two days later.

The doctor, by losing his temper and not insisting more determinedly, was just as foolish as Anthony was in his stubborn refusal. A calm and reasoned approach entails weighing the implications of both actions. You have to decide open-mindedly if the risk of an X ray outweighs that of developing an undiagnosed and possibly treatable disease. Doctors now are much better informed and careful about ordering X rays than they were 20 years ago. If you're nervous about the X ray, speak up and listen carefully to your doctor's reply. If you're pregnant, or think you might be, tell the doctor *and* the X-ray technician. They will shield your pelvis during the process.

Laboratory Tests

Depending on your situation, the doctor may order some laboratory work. In addition to a urinalysis, which can point to any one of a large number of conditions, you may have blood samples drawn. Many individuals find this experience upsetting and painful, but it is useful in detecting anemia or infections. It can also establish the presence of immunoglobulin E (IgE), a strong indicator of an allergic base for your asthma. A tuberculin skin test, to determine if you have been exposed to tuberculosis, may be administered because this disease, once a rarity, is making a determined comeback. Finally, the doctor will consider and discuss with you the possibility and advisability of having allergy skin tests. Skin tests and other tests for allergies — and their place in diagnosing asthma — are discussed in detail in Chapter 5.

CHOOSING A PHYSICIAN

There are a number of things to look for in a physician and they apply regardless of the source of your medical care — independent, private physicians or a large health maintenance organization. Most important, you should feel comfortable with your physician and have solid reason to believe that he or she is well trained and competent. When you first call for an appointment, inquire where the doctor received his or her training. You may find the following guidelines useful:

1. *Is the doctor a graduate of an American medical school?*
Levels of training and standards of performance demanded in medical education vary greatly around the world. U.S. schools enforce fairly consistent standards, and their graduates perform better in medical qualifying examinations.

2. *What is the doctor's specialty, and does he or she have board certification to back it up?*
Upon graduating from medical school, the brand new doctor who has merely completed his medical school courses is awarded a license to practice "medicine and surgery." This occurs before undergoing any intensive clinical experience (internship) or specialized training (residency) and does not really signify that its holder is competent to practice. Having an M.D. degree alone does not qualify its holder to go out and practice allergy or any other specialty.

There are a number of medical groups that have acquired the special training and background that qualify them to treat asthma. These are pediatricians, internists, chest or pulmonary physicians, and allergists. Depending on your age, your first asthma visit should probably be to a pediatrician (for children or youth) or an internist (for adolescents and older). Most patients with asthma are adequately treated by pediatricians and internists. Make sure, however, that your prospective physician is board certified in pediatrics or internal medicine. If the receptionist or office nurse does not know about certification, the doctor is probably not certified. Insist until you get a definite yes or no answer to the question of board certification.

You can also start with a family practitioner (not the same as the old-time general practitioner), who has had special training in family medicine. Family practitioners can manage most routine medical problems efficiently and competently, but for serious asthmatic symptoms you should be referred to an internist, a pediatrician, or either a chest physician or an allergist for consultation.

3. *Choose a doctor when you are healthy.*
Too often, people moving to a new town put off finding someone to take care of them. Then, when they get sick, they no longer have the freedom or time to choose carefully. For them it's the emergency room and pot luck. It is also hard on a new doctor to examine you during a crisis, having to make decisions without knowing you, your history, or your physical exam results.

If you are new in town and have no idea where to go, call the county medical society or the nearest medical school. Ask what internists or family practitioners are located near your work or home. Then, check on board certification and training, as discussed earlier. Shop around. Ask the receptionist for names of neighbors who are patients of that doctor and solicit their opinions about the quality and cost of the care they receive. Visit the doctor's office and arrange to have your medical records transferred. If you are not satisfied with the doctor's attitude or work schedule, then it's time to go shopping again.

4. *Having a family practitioner, an internist, or a pediatrician in addition to any specialists you require.*

Just because you have asthma does not mean that you should only see an allergist or a chest physician. Have someone available who cares about your whole body, someone you can consult about your headache or your infected toe, someone who can answer questions about how good a job your allergist may be doing.

5. *Choose a doctor who asks about the "healthy things" you are doing, who cares about prevention, not just doctoring you when you are sick.*

A healthy life-style depends on prevention. Your doctor should want to see you periodically, even if only once every year or two, for a physical examination. Select someone who inquires about your diet and your use of vitamins, who cares about your weight and your smoking and drinking habits. These questions point to a doctor who cares about maintaining your good health, not just treating your disease.

6. *Do you feel comfortable with your doctor?*

This is by far the most important feature. Doctors are people too. They get sick and have to see doctors themselves. They can be hurried, harried, and sometimes unsure of themselves. A good bedside manner in the old days was largely a matter of knowing you as a person. It meant being willing to stop, listen, and respond honestly and fully to your questions. This openness should exist between you and your physician. When it is absent you should try to establish it. Physicians sometimes do not question or probe; if they are brusque and devote less time to the human side of illness — the confusion, the fear, the misunderstanding, the pain — then they are not providing the best possible medical care.

When to Consult a
Chest Physician or Allergist

Both chest physicians and allergists are thoroughly trained and experienced in the care of patients with asthma. Yet, surprisingly, the chest physician will often express negative opinions about the allergist, while the allergist may declare that the chest physician has it all wrong. The animosity between these two groups of physicians has much to do with their different opinions about the value of skin tests and allergy shots. Most chest physicians believe that asthma is best managed by medications and that allergy shots have little if any valid role in treatment. Allergists, on the other hand, think that skin tests and allergy shots may be extremely important and helpful in caring for asthma.

If you have extrinsic asthma (see Chapter 1), you should certainly consult an allergist at some point in your care. On the other hand, if your asthma is intrinsic, with no seasonal aggravation and no obvious pollen or environmental triggering factors, a workup by an allergist is unnecessary. Good allergists recognize this and — following history, physical exam, and perhaps skin tests — will return the non-extrinsic asthmatics to the care of their original internist or pediatrician or perhaps refer them directly to a chest physician.

The matter of referral brings up another important point. Choose a physician who will not hesitate to seek a second opinion or to obtain special consultative help for you. It is your life and your health. If your physician has the kind of ego that makes it hard to seek help and guidance from other physicians, then you should get somebody else.

Other Factors to Consider

Coverage

People get sick 24 hours a day. When you seek out a physician, find out if round-the-clock coverage is provided. If your doctor relies on the Emergency Room and the doctor on call there for backup, then find someone else. Good physicians offer full coverage for their patients. While it is impossible for physicians to be on call 24 hours a day for all of their patients, they can work out sharing arrangements with similar groups of specialty physicians. Thus a group of internists may share "on call" with one another; so may a group of allergists. This assures that their patients will be adequately covered in an emergency. It also means that the physician on call has access to your medical records and knows where to reach your physician, should that be necessary.

Fees and Hours

A physician needs to earn a living like any other individual, but money should not be his or her sole reason for treating you. We are weary and a bit distrustful of physicians who require cash payments up front before treatment. Money is important to patients too, and you should not be afraid to ask the doctor what the charges are and what mode of billing and payment applies. If the doctor gets touchy about money and treats you like a second-class citizen because you are concerned about money, then you are seeing the wrong person. If the doctor refuses to accept you as a patient because your resources are inadequate or your insurance coverage is unacceptable, ask to be recommended to someone else. Good physicians accept responsibility for finding alternative care for people they are themselves unwilling to treat — especially when the reasons are purely economic ones.

Don't choose a doctor with 10 patients in the office, all of them with one o'clock appointments. Such a practitioner will probably be too harried, rushing from one patient to another, to give you the time and personal attention you need and deserve.

What about a Second Opinion?

Second opinions are a way of life in medicine. If you want a second opinion, ask your doctor to recommend someone. Sometimes you may be referred to an associate in the same office; often you may be sent to a medical school or a large clinic. However, do it openly and seek your own doctor's cooperation. Don't go around "doctor shopping," looking for good news. It helps the second doctor if you bring all your records — after all, you paid for them — and can legitimately insist they be provided. Without them, it's like starting to run the race all over again from the beginning. Time and money are wasted.

> Dr. Francis has been Pam's physician for more than 20 years. In fact, he delivered her. Pam has been seeing him for asthma for nearly 10 years. She is concerned that the treatment he recommends for her asthma may not be the most current or the best. Generally, she feels well, but on occasion she has bouts of wheezing which are not as readily controlled as she would like. She wants to ask Dr. Francis to recommend someone for a second opinion but is afraid of offending him. Instead, she goes across town and sees a specialist, Dr. Gray. She does not plan to give the specialist Dr. Francis's name, but somehow it slips into the conversation. The specialist reviews the medication she is on and makes some minor changes and suggestions. About six weeks later Pam sees Dr. Francis for her regular checkup. She is surprised when he says he is glad that Pam saw Dr. Gray. He explains that the specialist had been courteous enough to give him a phone call and had sent a letter describing what his results and recommendations were.

> Dr. Oliver is an outstanding chest physician, one with enough board certificates and diplomas to fill an entire wall. He also has an ego to match. At a medical conference, a colleague, Dr. Madison, told Dr. Oliver that he had seen Lou R., one of his patients. In fact, Lou had called and made an appointment without a referral. Lou also requested that Dr. Madison not inform Dr. Oliver. Dr. Madison thought Lou was being too concerned about Dr. Oliver's feelings and said that he would mention it the next time they happened to meet. Dr. Oliver's reaction to the disclosure astounded Dr. Madison. Dr. Oliver went into a rage. He said that he did not want his patient seen by other doctors unless he approved it. Then, to make matters worse, he was extremely rude to Lou on his next visit. Unfortunately, Lou, like many others, considers doctors to be above reproach and continues to see him.

BEING A GOOD PATIENT

In this book we emphasize how you must take charge of your asthma and be ultimately responsible for yourself and your disease. To do this you obviously need information, understanding, and the willingness to look, listen, and make decisions, some of them risky. A very important part of being able to take charge of your asthma is being a responsible patient. Be prepared to describe everything to your doctor as carefully and in as much detail as you possibly can. When you consult your doctor, write down what bothers you before you get there. Be specific. Often the doctor may start out the conversation by asking you how everyone is at home and how you are enjoying the weather. The doctor is doing this to relax you, not invite you to chat. This may divert attention from your problem and get in the way of talking about what is troubling you, which should be the focus of your visit.

There are a number of specific questions that you should be prepared to ask, and to note the answers. For asthmatics, they might include the following:

1. What are the types of drugs being prescribed?
2. What are the harmful side effects or risks of these drugs?
3. How soon should the drugs work?
4. How long should I take the drugs?
5. Should I call the doctor if the treatment does not help? How soon?
6. When should I see the doctor again?
7. Is a second opinion appropriate in my case? Will the doctor recommend someone?

Establishing an honest, open relationship with your (or your child's) doctor makes coping with the illness considerably easier. It will help you both to weather the crises and enjoy the periods of remission.

Breathing and Other Exercises to Ease Asthma Attacks

GETTING RID OF MUCUS

During an asthma attack the goblet cells (see Chapter 1) that line the airways increase their production of mucus drastically. When this sticky, tenacious mucus lodges in your airways it makes breathing even more difficult. Sometimes it gets so bad that asthmatics literally drown in their own phlegm.

There is nothing you can do to affect the production of mucus, but there are simple and effective steps you can take to keep it thin and easy to move. Also, by knowing what to do, you can get it up and out of your lungs.

To keep mucus from getting dangerously thick and clingy, you must increase your fluid intake, drinking at least two full glasses of water four times a day, increasing your overall daily fluid consumption to 60 ounces (two quarts) or more. Water is best. Stay away from juices, milk, or other beverages, which carry the possibility of allergic complications and do not get absorbed by the body any faster. Some physicians recommend "sports drinks" like Gatorade because they contain a purportedly ideal balance of salts and vitamins. Their superiority to plain, unadulterated water has not been established.

Getting the mucus *out* is a bit more difficult. However, it can be done readily enough provided you devote time to it, get help, and overcome any scruples you have about hawking up phlegm. What you will be doing, in fact, is getting the phlegm *down* and out, because the exercises we recommend involve a series of postures where the chest and torso are higher than your head. The mucus, aided by gravity and gentle tapping, will be dislodged and ooze out of the airways. To do this you will need a stiff, wedge-shaped bolster a couple of feet square and at least 4 – 6 inches higher at one end. Such bolsters can be obtained from the bedding department of most larger department stores or sleep shops and cost under $20.

Lie on the bolster, belt line at the high end, head on the floor at the low end, back down (Figure 11a), then each side down, then face down (Figure 11b).

In each position have someone tap the uppermost part of your chest gently and steadily with their stiffened fingers (Figure 11c). This will loosen the clinging mucus and speed its outward flow. The tapping helps greatly and can be fun too. If there is no one around to assist, a hand-held vibrator will produce the same results. Stay in each position from three to five minutes, and do the mucus clearing twice a day. If you schedule one session just before going to bed, it will help you sleep.

FIGURE 11   Exercises for Clearing Mucus

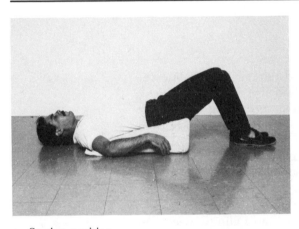

a. Supine position

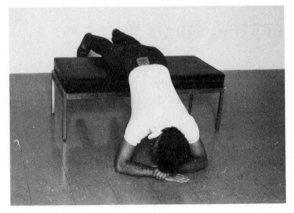

b. Prone position

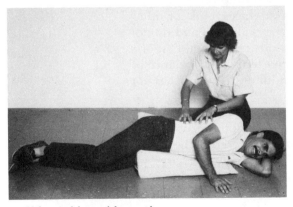

c. Side position with tapping

IMPROVING BREATHING

You can greatly reduce the severity of asthmatic attacks if you practice breathing. "Why should I practice breathing?" you may ask. "I've been breathing all my life."

True enough. Yet, unless you are a serious athlete or an aerobics practitioner, chances are good that you have never used about one-third of your lung capacity. This backlog of brand-new lung tissue can really help you minimize the effects of your twitchy airways and bronchospasm and make your medication much more effective in controlling them.

There are three different kinds of exercises that will improve your breathing. The first kind helps you involve your diaphragm in the process of breathing — something that most people don't do.

Diaphragmatic Breathing Exercises

1. Locate your diaphragm (which is a large, powerful muscle) by putting your hands on your stomach between your navel and the rib cage. (See Figure 12a.)
2. Keeping your hands on the diaphragm, take a deep breath. If you are using your diaphragm, your hands will be pushed forward. Then exhale; your hands should now move inward.
3. Once you get to the point where you can move the diaphragm, practice diaphragmatic breathing four times a day for three or four minutes each time. Keep your hands on the diaphragm always and do the breathing exercise standing for one minute, sitting for one minute, and reclining on your back for one minute.
4. When, after a week or so, diaphragmatic breathing gets to be automatic, add this exercise: lie on your back, and place a weight (4–5 pounds of books is about right) on your diaphragm. Breathe in deeply, using your diaphragm, and then exhale slowly. Repeat this exercise 10 or a dozen times twice daily. This will strengthen the diaphragm. (See Figure 12b.)

Breathing Exercises

A second kind of breathing exercise helps you expand your rib cage and get those unused lung cells into action.

1. Lock your hands behind your neck and press your elbows back as you inhale. Hold your breath a few seconds then exhale while bringing your elbows together in front of you. (This exercise can be done sitting, standing, or lying down.) Repeat 10 times, twice a day. (See Figures 13a and 13b.)
2. Seat yourself upright on a straight-backed chair. Raise your arms high while inhaling, then slowly bend forward and exhale slowly. Your

hands should touch the floor. Repeat 10 times twice a day. (See Figures 13c and 13d.)

3. Seat yourself upright. Put one hand on your stomach and extend the other arm out horizontally away from the body as you inhale deeply. Exhale slowly and, as you do this, bring the hand of the extended arm to the opposite shoulder. Repeat, alternating positions of hands, 10 times twice daily. (See Figures 13e and 13f.)

These exercises are all designed to increase airway capacity. Somewhat the same effect can be achieved by acquiring and using an inspiratory muscle trainer, a small plastic device which, by slightly obstructing the flow of air, causes extra effort to be exerted in inspiration. It is less conspicuous than the exercises and is an effective way to improve breathing and respiratory reserve.

FIGURE 12   Diaphragmatic Breathing Exercises

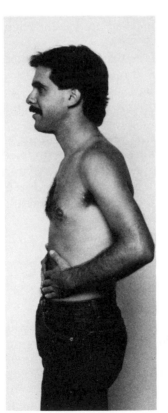

a. Standing position: exhale

b. Supine with weights

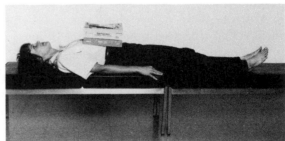

Bronchial Exercise

As you know, the bronchial tubes have walls of smooth muscle, and it is this muscle that contracts and causes wheezing and shortness of breath. The bronchial walls can be strengthened and made more resistant to spasm through the third exercise.

Clench your fingers to make a closed cylinder of your hand (the kind you make when your hands are cold and you want to blow on them to warm them). Try to make the cylinder as tight as possible. Blow into it,

FIGURE 13 Other Breathing Exercises

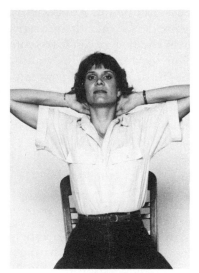

a. Elbow flex: inhale

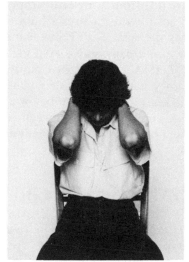

b. Elbow flex: exhale

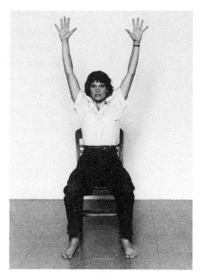

c. "In praise": inhale

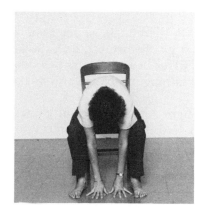

d. "In praise": exhale

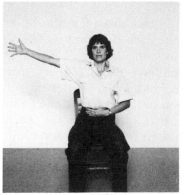

e. Arm to shoulder: inhale

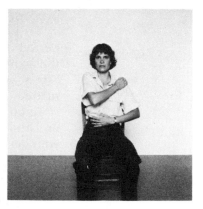

f. Arm to shoulder: exhale

remove from your mouth, inhale, blow again with increasing force. Do this for a minute or two, three times daily.

These breathing exercises altogether will take less than an hour of your time, per day. Yet, if you do them regularly — and they can be done almost anyplace, anytime — your lung capacity, your muscle tone, and your resistance to asthmatic bronchospasm will be phenomenally increased. It's well worth the effort.

Monitoring Respiratory Status

To see an objective record of your progress, obtain a peak expiratory flow meter (Figure 14) from a medical supply house, as listed in Appendix H. If your physician writes a prescription for this device, health insurance should defray the cost. A PEF meter measures the flow of air from your lungs. Blow into it daily and keep a log of your performance, as you did with the ASTHMA FINDER in Chapter 5. Use this device to monitor your respiratory status; it may alert you to the need for medication *before* an acute attack. A measurement below about 80 percent of your best PEF indicates that you may need more medication. If you score below 50 percent, take a bronchodilator immediately and call your physician.

SPECIAL EXERCISES FOR CHILDREN

Even in older children and adults there is a strong tendency not to adhere to a regular program of breathing exercises. In young children (those under eight) this tendency becomes almost irresistible. However, the inherent boredom and lack of immediate payoff can be countered if the activity is made pleasurable and if tangible rewards are built into the process.

To provide this sort of incentive, you, the parent, must set aside a period of time each day for practice, such as just before bedtime. Make the activity as gamelike, as rewarding, and as free of coercion as possible. Stress, as we have noted, can intensify breathing problems and make matters worse rather than better.

In addition to the exercises cited above, here are a number of games, or contests, that can engage the attention and sustain the interest of younger children from age 3 onward.

1. Get (or have your child help you make) an ordinary pinwheel. Mount the pinwheel on a stick — a piece of ¼-inch doweling works well for this purpose. Hold the pinwheel in front of the child about 6 inches from the mouth. Have the child blow the pinwheel and record how many seconds it is kept in motion in one sustained breath. Repeat five times and record the total time for the session on an activity record

(like an attendance or achievement chart), which can be made and posted on the wall of the child's room. Praise the effort and make a point of noting and rewarding improvement, such as with small toys, books, and additional privileges.

2. Follow the same procedure as with the pinwheel for a single piece of toilet tissue held to the wall by a sustained breath. Scoring and reward procedure are the same as for exercise 1 above (Figure 15a).

FIGURE 14   Peak Expiratory Flow Meter in Use

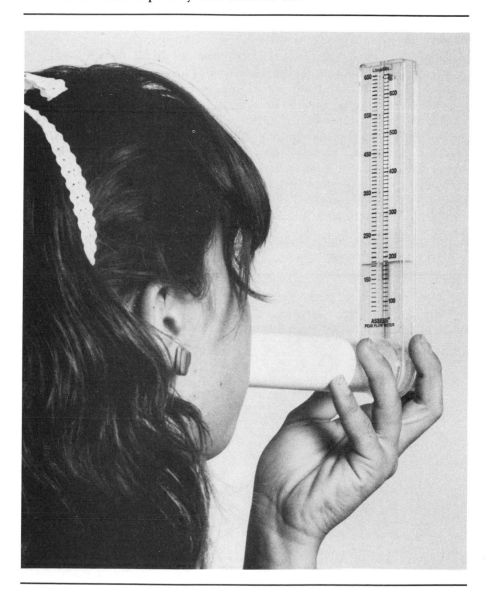

3. Put a small amount of detergent and water into a mixing bowl. Give the child a straw and record the length of time the child is able to produce bubbles by blowing through the straw held in the fluid (Figure 15b). Record the longest time the child is able to sustain one breath. (An average score for the first session is 5 seconds; work to improve.)

4. Record the amount of time the child is able to sustain a continuous, audible sound on a musical toy or instrument like a whistle or a harmonica. (Number of trials here may depend on parental tolerance for noise.)

5. Balloon blowing is good for children ages six or older. (Children under six have been known to aspirate balloons.) Here, measure the size to which an easily inflated balloon can be blown with one continuous breath.

6. An almost endless variety of respiration-improving games can be devised using Ping-Pong balls. For example, set up an obstacle course or maze on a kitchen or dining table (books are good for this purpose) and see how far the child is able to propel the ball through the maze with one sustained breath; or get into the act yourself by stationing yourself across the table from the child, ball positioned in the center. On signal, try to blow the ball off the table on the opponent's side. (You do not have to win except once in a while; loser has to retrieve the ball. Repeat five times; record number of wins for each player.)

7. There are also versions of bowls or boccie that can be worked out by using different colored balls on a (relatively) smooth floor surface. Place the target ball at some distance from the starting point. Players

FIGURE 15   Children's Breathing Improvement Games

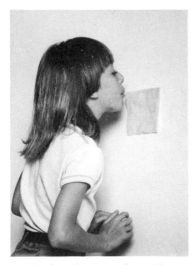 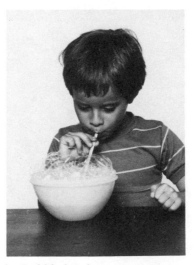 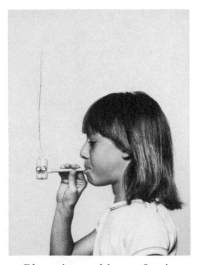

a. Pinning tissue to the wall   b. Bubble bowl   c. Blow pipe and loop of string

try to get their own ball closest to the target by blowing it. (As breathing improves, distances can be increased.)

8. Another form of exercise is available in the form of a toy that can be found in some toy shops. It consists of a pipe which, when blown through, will create a column of moving air which will support a Ping-Pong ball or hold a loop of string (Figure 15c). Here the record of progress would be the longest time the ball is kept aloft in five tries. Candles can also be used in games to improve and sustain peak flow.

The resourceful parent or sibling can come up with many other ways of encouraging the asthmatic child to improve lung capacity without making it seem like a chore. As a general rule, depend heavily on honest praise; steer clear of food rewards. Participation and enthusiasm will not flag if it is made a regular, fun part of the daily routine, if it is reinforced by sincere praise and tangible rewards or tokens, and if there is a clear record of progress.

15 The Use of Drugs to Prevent or Relieve Asthma Symptoms

PRESCRIPTION ASTHMA MEDICATIONS

Several medications, used appropriately, keep asthma symptoms from appearing or relieve them when they are present. There are five general classes of these medications: beta agonists, topical steroids, theophylline, cromolyn, and oral steroids.

These drugs must be ordered for you by your doctor. Each has a special place in the armamentarium of prescription drugs and, if taken properly, can be enormously helpful in abating or controlling symptoms. At the end of the chapter we cover many of the over-the-counter (OTC), or nonprescription, drugs that are available for relieving asthma symptoms.

Some of these drugs can only be taken orally. Some can be taken orally or can be inhaled directly into the lungs for more immediate relief. There are three widely used methods of taking medication by inhalation. The first method is by metered-dose inhalation using a hand-held canister of aerolized medication. The second is by a process called nebulization using a home air compressor. The third is by use of a device called a Rotahaler. Relief depends on understanding how, why, and when to use these medications.

Beta Agonists

Beta agonists are the mainstay of treatment for patients with asthma. These drugs (Table 11) are most commonly and most effectively administered by means of a metered, hand-held aerosol canister. Activating the canister releases a puff of drug-saturated aerosol which is carried directly to the airways and which acts to ease or relax the muscle spasm. This direct action of muscle relaxation quells the symptoms much more rapidly than any other class of drugs. A canister can be conveniently carried in the pocket or purse.

Aerosols for the treatment of asthma have been on the market for more than three decades. The effectiveness of aerosols depends very much on knowing how to use them:

1. DO NOT OVERUSE. Take one or two inhalations every four hours, no more than 12 puffs a day, unless your doctor has given you specific instructions to the contrary.
2. Be alert for side effects, including irregular or rapid heartbeat, nervousness, muscle tremors, nausea, vomiting, dizziness, weakness, sweating, or chest pain. If any of these appear, discontinue and proceed immediately to the emergency room.
3. Do not use these drugs unless you have specifically discussed them with your physician. If you have high blood pressure, hyperthyroidism, or cardiac disease, these drugs may not be right for you.

How to Use a Metered Aerosol

1. Shake inhaler.
2. Begin inhalation and, at the same time, place aerosol just in front of your mouth and release a properly aimed puff of aerosol. (Aerosol should go straight to the large airways; it should not hit the back of the throat. See Figure 16.)
3. Inhale at a moderate rate with open mouth.
4. Hold breath for five seconds.
5. Exhale.
6. Repeat steps 2–5, *one time only*, if necessary.
7. If you still have problems using metered-dose inhalers, consult your doctor, who may prescribe use of a spacing device such as Inspir-Ease.

Even children as young as four can be taught to use metered aerosols. Their parents can skillfully press on the canister of the inhaler while the child takes a breath. In both adults and children, however, if the canister is aimed incorrectly, the medicine is likely to land uselessly on the roof of the mouth or the tongue. If not coordinated with inhaling, it will fail to reach the lungs. Previous studies in children using inhalers have revealed that as many as one-third of them are not using the device properly and are losing most of its significant benefits. To overcome these deficiencies, two other delivery systems have been developed.

The first and older form of remedying this deficiency entails the use of a "spacer." A spacer is simply a device that makes it easier to deliver the drug to your lungs by coordinating timing, aiming, and breathing. A

TABLE 11 Prescription Beta Agonist Medications

Brand Name	Advantages	Disadvantages
Metered Hand-Held Aerosols Isoproterenol (Isuprel, Medihaler-Iso)	None known	Very short duration of action, 1 hour; causes tremors, rapid heart beat
Bronkosol	Rapid onset of action	Very short duration of action, 1 hour; causes tremors, rapid heart beat
Metaproterenol (Alupent, Metaprel)	Rapid onset of action	Short duration of action, 2–4 hours
Albuterol (Proventil, Ventolin)	Rapid onset of action	Duration of action, 3–5 hours
Terbutaline (Brethaire)	Rapid onset of action	Duration of action, 4–6 hours; "tolerance" to drug or decreased effectiveness after prolonged use has been reported
Bitolterol Mesylate (Tornalate)	Long duration of action	Takes up to 30 minutes to work
Pirbuterol Acetate (Maxair)	Long duration of action; comes with its own built-in spacing device	Duration of action, 5–6 hours
Rotahalers Ventolin	Rapid onset of action	Effective for young children and those who cannot use metered-dose inhalers
Oral Preparations (short-acting) Isuprel Metaproterenol (Alupent, Metaprel) 10, 20 mg tabs, 10 mg/5 ml liquid Terbutaline (Brethine, Bricayl), 2–5, 5 mg, 1 mg/ml liquid Albuterol (Proventil, Ventolin), 2, 4 mg tabs, 2 mg/5 ml liquid		All oral preparations are less effective than proper use of metered aerosol preparation of the same drug
Oral Preparation (extended release) Proventil repetabs, 4 mg		Less effective than metered aerosol
Solutions for Nebulization Alupent	Rapid onset of action	Tremors, rapid heart beat
Ventolin (Proventil)		Tremors, rapid heart beat

cheap, effective spacing device can be had from the cardboard cylinder found within a roll of toilet paper or a disposable paper cup. The patient activates the inhaler to release the drug into the spacing device, then inhales slowly from the spacer. Most of the time this works quite well. However, we prefer and recommend that you use the Inspir-Ease. This device costs approximately $16. It consists of a mouthpiece and an inflatable bag. The mouthpiece is made of plastic and should last for up to a year. The bag should be changed often; bags are generally sold in packages of 10. (Many parents have found that the bags can be washed, air-dried, and used again. This will likely work two or three times but does not offer a permanent solution because the bags develop holes and there is always the chance of bacterial contamination.)

FIGURE 16 Typical Metered Hand-Held Beta Agonist Aerosol

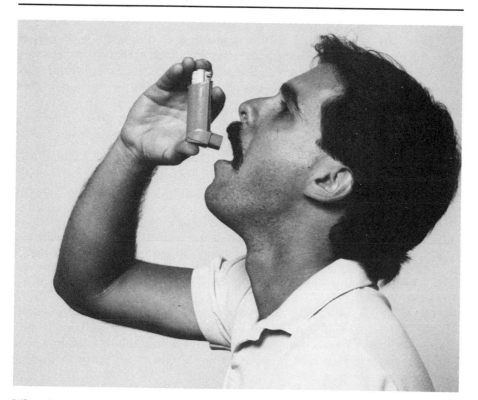

When in use the head is held back to open up airways. The canister is placed 1–2 inches in front of the open mouth. This enables the drug to enter the airways and reduces the chance of it hitting the back of the throat.

The newest metered-dose inhaler, a drug called Maxair, comes with its own, built-in spacing device. This is simply a larger mouthpiece which allows for more effective delivery. Users don't have to buy or create their own spacer.

Another form of drug delivery system which can be extremely useful is called the Rotahaler. It consists of a 3-inch cylinder of plastic. Inside the cylinder is a little pin and propeller. The beta agonist drug comes as a capsule containing a powder. The capsule is put inside the propeller shaft where the pin punctures it. When you inhale, you breathe in the powder inside the capsule. This is an extremely effective and simple system for very young children to master. It delivers drugs as efficiently as a metered-dose inhaler, and studies of children have shown it to be extremely useful. Often young children will pre-load their Rotahaler, put it on their night table, and take and use it during the night if they wake up wheezing. Although most people have found that the Rotahaler does not offer significant advantages over metered-dose inhalers, such devices are a useful alternative for children or other people with poor eye-hand coordination. (Other means of dry-powder delivery have been more extensively used in Europe and Asia.)

There have been reports of bizarre and tragic complications associated with the use of metered-dose inhalers. Always take care to avoid inhaling foreign objects. All the metered-dose inhalers, with the exception of Maxair, come with a cap. Sometimes users forget to remove the cap. When they press on the canister, the cap is propelled into the mouth — even, on occasion, into the airways. The Maxair inhaler avoids this problem because its hinged cap actually folds up and becomes part of the mouthpiece. With all inhalers, including Maxair, foreign objects — coins, dirt, and other small objects — may lodge in the mouthpiece.

> Dr. Fields really gets into his gardening. There are times when he's up to his knees in soil, mud, and leaves. One day while gardening, his chest became a little tight, so he reached into his overalls for his inhaler. Without bothering to look, he popped off the cap and sprayed a whole mouthful of dirt into his mouth and airways. It took 15 minutes and considerable anguished coughing for him to spew out all the matter he had inhaled. The dirt had found its way from garden to pocket to mouthpiece and finally into Dr. Fields.

Almost all of these beta agonists are available in pill or liquid form. However, we prefer the metered-dose aerosols or the Rotahaler to pills because of their rapid action, effectiveness, and immediate availability. In addition, the side effects of rapid heart rate, tremors, and muscle shaking are worse using pills or liquid.

Finally, we should mention that Alupent and Ventolin (Proventil) are both available in solution by nebulization via a home air compressor. This is by far the most effective way of delivering beta agonists. For people with moderate to severe asthma or for very young children, the use of home air compressors is strongly recommended. Their features and use are discussed later in this chapter.

Topical Steroids

In the past, steroids, drugs in the cortisone family, were reserved for individuals with very severe asthma, especially those who were or had at one time been hospitalized. These drugs carry major and dangerous side effects and, if taken for long periods of time, cause the body to bloat and gain weight. They induce water retention and elevate blood pressure. They can also make the skin become thin and are known to cause osteoporosis, or thinning of the bones. They can cause easy bruising. Cortisone can also make the body more susceptible to infection and is known to cause cataracts. Use of corticosteroids has also been associated with degeneration of the joints, particularly a syndrome called avascular necrosis of the hip (AVN). Because of these drastic side effects, cortisone is a drug which, when administered orally, even in small doses, should be used carefully and only when necessary.

However, there has been a revolution in the use of cortisone. One way individuals who really need daily administration of cortisone can dodge its side effects is to take a special topical preparation of cortisone (Table 12). These forms of cortisone are not absorbed into the body in significant amounts. The first of these topical preparations is beclomethasone, sold under the brand names Vanceril and Beclovent. Beclomethasone is administered using a metered-dose inhaler much like beta agonists so that, if properly taken several times per day, the drug acts only on the lungs. Unless beclomethasone is used more often than recommended, it does not produce the dangerous side effects associated with oral steroids.

Two other topical steroids are now also available. One is called AeroBid. This has the advantages of beclomethasone and the additional feature of requiring dosages only twice daily. However, it has a disagreeable taste and can induce nausea and upset stomach in many users. In our experience, most people are unable to tolerate it. Most recently, a topical steroid called Azmacort was released. Azmacort is as effective as beclomethasone. However, it has an enormous advantage over the other topical steroids in that it is supplied with a built-in spacing device. This makes delivery of the drug much more efficient. For many people, the use of Azmacort has dramatically changed their lives for the better (see Figure 17).

TABLE 12   Topical Steroid Preparations

Brand Name	Advantages	Disadvantages
Beclomethasone (Beclovent, Vanceril)	Has been used successfully for more than 10 years	Has no spacer
AeroBid	Effective when given only twice a day	Bad taste; often induces nausea
Azmacort	Comes with a spacer which helps delivery	None

Five years ago, the use of topical steroids was reserved for individuals who had not been helped by conventional therapy: beta agonists, theophylline, and Intal. However, more recent studies suggest that drugs like Azmacort have few side effects, can be tolerated for long periods of time, and are an appropriate primary medication for the treatment of many asthmatics. Azmacort has become a primary or secondary stage of treat-

FIGURE 17   Use of Azmacort Spacer

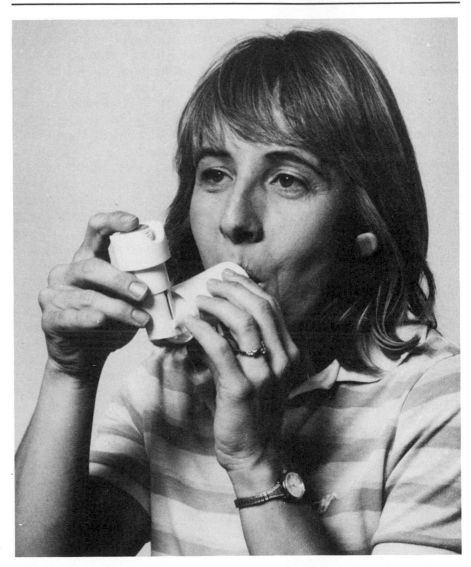

Azmacort, a topical steroid, comes with a spacer, which helps with the delivery of the drug.

ment for many with asthma. The results have been gratifying and we expect that use of drugs like Azmacort will continue to increase as newer and more effective agents are developed. For patients who rely on more than one inhaler, we recommend that first the beta agonist be used, then the topical steroid.

Theophyllines

Theophyllines are drugs that are chemically very similar to caffeine. Indeed, it has been known for centuries that many asthmatics show significant improvement upon drinking a cup of strong coffee. Theophyllines used to be the first line of treatment for asthma. However, the side effects of theophylline are unpleasant and can include nausea, vomiting, and central nervous system stimulation. There have been several deaths reported among children who used theophylline. Although theophylline remains an important ancillary drug in the management of asthma for most asthmatics, it should be used only after trying beta agonists and inhaled steroids first.

Theophyllines relax bronchial smooth muscle, thus opening up airways and making breathing easier. When taken properly, theophylline keeps wheezing from developing in most mild to moderate asthmatics and allows them to lead a more comfortable, normal life. However, it may be several hours before theophylline begins to relieve the symptoms. It can irritate the stomach and, in large doses, has many of caffeine's undesirable side effects. It is a strong stimulant, can make sleep difficult, and increases urine output. In rare cases it may even be toxic; high dosages can trigger nausea, vomiting, tremors, rapid heart rate, convulsions, and even death.

Taking the correct amount of theophylline is crucial. Proper dosage depends on body size and must be carefully calculated by your doctor. Dosage may also be affected by your age, other medicines you may be taking, and any underlying illnesses. Even then, there are sometimes significant differences in reactions between like-sized individuals. Therefore, physicians order a blood test several days after starting the drug to ascertain how much theophylline is in your blood. If your asthma is not responding to theophylline, see your doctor — don't double your dose!

Theophylline is usually prescribed for chronic moderate to severe asthmatics, and comes in five forms: liquid, chewable tablets, short-acting pills, long-acting pills and "beaded" capsules, and very long-acting pills.

Liquid forms of theophylline (Table 13) have a disagreeable taste. At one time they represented the only way that theophylline could be given to small children who were unable to swallow pills. We do not recommend theophylline in liquid form because children either refuse to swallow it or (if they do) often vomit it back up. This means that a large quantity has to be swallowed to reach a therapeutically effective dose.

"Theophylline Chewable" is intended for children who cannot swallow pills. It, too, tastes extremely bitter and in our experience is not satisfactory. For young children who cannot swallow pills, we recommend the beaded-capsule method.

The third type of theophylline comes in the form of a "short-acting" pill (Table 13). Formerly it was the major way to prescribe theophylline. These short-acting preparations are rapidly degraded in the body and have to be taken every four to six hours to maintain round-the-clock protection. Many asthmatics are not helped greatly by these pills because of this short duration of action. In addition, most people find it difficult to stick to a strict medication schedule. As a result theophylline levels in the blood may fluctuate widely. This often causes problems at night. Finally, the metabolism of theophylline — the rate at which it is absorbed in the body — varies for a number of reasons. Many drugs, including the common antibiotic erythromycin, alter the survival time of theophyllines. Smoking, as well as heart, liver, and kidney disease, can also affect the metabolism of the drug. For these reasons, asthmatics often fail to get as much relief out of the short-acting theophyllines as they should. We seldom recommend them.

The fourth type of theophylline is a "long-acting" form, either a pill or a bead-filled time-release capsule (Table 14). These preparations are manufactured to increase their survival time in the body and thus to make it easier to achieve round-the-clock protection. They are generally effective when taken two to three times a day. Many people take them at bedtime for nighttime protection. For children who have difficulty swallowing pills, the beaded capsule can be opened and the beads mixed with soft foods like applesauce or yogurt and administered in that way. One caveat is that absorption of beads is often erratic in young children, especially children under six. If it works, however, it is infinitely preferable to the disagreeable-tasting liquid form. When taken regularly (with careful initial monitoring of the blood to determine the optimal dose and to detect potentially dangerous side effects), long-acting theophylline keeps wheezing from developing in most mild to moderate asthmatics and allows them to lead a much more comfortable and normal life.

The fifth preparation of theophylline is a new and purportedly very long-acting form that is said to be effective when given only once a day. The efficacy of these drugs (Theo 24, Uniphyl) is often uneven and variable. Their effects are particularly unpredictable in very young patients. We prefer not to use them until more reliable manufacturing processes are developed that will turn out a dependable, one-dose-per-day product.

Cromolyn (Intal)

Cromolyn sodium, a synthetic chemical originally isolated from an Egyptian weed, is also used to control or ward off symptoms in chronic asthmatics with moderate to severe symptoms. In the United States it is marketed as Intal.

TABLE 13   Short-Acting Liquid and Immediate-Release Tablet Theopyllines*

Brand Name	
Liquid	
Accurbron	
Aerolate oral syrup solution	
Aminophylline oral liquid	Contains 79% theophylline
Aquaphylline syrup	
Asmalix elixir	
Choledyl elixir	Contains 64% theophylline
Choledyl syrup, pediatric	Contains 64% theophylline
Dilor elixir	Contains dyphylline
Elixophyllin elixir	
Elixophyllin oral solution	
Lanophyllin elixir	
Luphyllin elixir	Contains dyphylline
Oxtriphylline elixir	Contains 64% theophylline
Oxtuphylline syrup, pediatric	Contains 64% theophylline
Slo-Phyllin syrup	
Theoclean-80 syrup	
Theolair solution	
Theophylline elixir	
Theophylline oral solution	
Theostat-80 syrup	

All have a disagreeable taste. It is difficult to establish effective levels of theophylline in children with any of these liquid preparations.

Tablet	
Aminophylline	100, 200 mg tablets (contains 70% theophylline)
Bronkodyl	100, 200 mg capsules
Choledyl	100, 200 mg tablets (contains oxtriphylline)
Dilor	200, 400 mg tablets (contains dyphylline)
Dyflex	200, 400 mg tablets (contains dyphylline)
Dyphylline	200, 400 mg tablets (contains dyphylline)
Elixophyllin	100, 200 mg capsules
Lyfylline	200, 400 mg tablets (contains dyphylline)
Marax	130 mg (also contains 25 mg ephedrine sulfate and 10 mg hydroxyzine HCl)
Neothylline	200, 400 mg tablets (contains dyphylline)
Oxtriphylline	100, 200 mg tablets (contains 64% theophylline)
Quibron-I Dividose	300 mg tablets
Theolair	125, 250 mg tablets
Theophylline	100, 200, 300 mg tablets

*Some of these short-acting theophyllines contain other drugs which are not generally recommended. Their use has been decreasing throughout the world.

TABLE 14   Long-Acting Theophylline Medications*

Theophylline	mg	Timed release (hours)
Sustained Release Capsules		
Aerolate	130, 260	8–12
Elixophyllin SR	125, 250	8–12
Slobid Gyrocaps	50, 75, 100, 125, 200, 300	8–12
Slophylline Gyrocaps	60, 125, 250	8–12
Theo-24	100, 200, 300	24
Theobid Jr. Duracaps	130	12
Theobid Duracaps	260	12
Theoclear LA	130, 260	12
Theodur Sprinkles	50, 75, 125, 200	12
Theospan-SR	130, 260	12
Theovent	125, 250	12
Sustained Release Tablets		
Constant-T	200, 300	8–12
Quibron-T/SR Dividose	300	8–12
Respbid	250, 500	8–12
Sustaine	100, 300	8–12
Theochron	100, 200, 300	12–24
Theodur	100, 200, 300, 450	8–24
Theolair-SR	200, 250, 300, 500	8–12
Theophylline SR	100, 200, 300	12–24
Theo-Sav	100, 200, 300	8–24
Theox	100, 200, 300	12–24
T-Phyl	200	8–12
Uniphyl	400	24
Oxtriphylline		
Choledyl-SA	400–600	12
Aminophylline		
Phyllocontin	225	12

*All achieve round-the-clock protection for most adults when taken 2 or 3 times a day.

Interestingly, in the 1960s when the drug first appeared on the market, it was heralded as the most effective asthma preventive available. Confidence in this prescription medication eroded quickly, however, partly because it sometimes seemed to make symptoms worse and partly because it is entirely a preventive measure and may need to be taken for several weeks before it begins to work. These features were not well understood then. In the past several years, and for good reasons, the drug has seen a major rebirth and is now widely used.

Cromolyn comes in two forms: as a metered-dose inhaler much like that of beta agonists and as a solution for nebulization. Cromolyn works entirely as a preventive. Thus, reaching in your pocket and using cromolyn when you start to wheeze is useless. Its effect is delayed, so it must be taken regularly and in the absence of symptoms, not just when you need it. For children who cannot use a cromolyn metered-dose inhaler, cromolyn may be administered in a home air compressor.

Cromolyn is extremely effective for exercise-induced asthma, helping hyperactive airways become less twitchy. Among its advantages are that unlike other asthma medications, it carries few and minor undesirable side effects and it does not interact with other drugs. We believe that cromolyn should be given a fair and serious trial — especially for a young child who is troubled with chronic moderate to severe extrinsic forms of asthma.

For people who take Intal and a beta agonist, we recommend that the beta agonist be taken first to help open the airways, followed by the Intal. A significant number of patients can control their asthma through use of the Intal inhaler alone. For most people, however, cromolyn remains an important but ancillary treatment.

Oral Steroids

Oral steroids are now reserved for individuals with severe, unremitting, or potentially life-threatening asthma. They should not be used daily unless the asthma is chronic and unresponsive to the other drugs outlined above. Steroids most often provide "pulse" or "burst" therapy for people with acute exacerbation of their asthma. Thus, someone with severe new-onset asthma, or someone in the midst of an acute episode, may receive a gradually tapering dose of Prednisone over a period of five days or more.

> Billy has severe asthma despite the use of beta agonists, Azmacort, and Intal. He developed influenza last winter and began to have uncontrollable wheezing. Billy's doctor, following his examination, prescribed Prednisone 60 mg for two days, then 40 mg × 2 days, then 20 mg × 2 days, then 10 mg. Billy then stopped the Prednisone. This several-day burst of steroids made his asthma tolerable and may have prevented hospitalization.

Once again, we stress that oral steroids, because of their serious and far-reaching side effects, should not be used routinely.

Combination Drugs

Once it was popular to prescribe pills that contained two or even three different ingredients. These pills are now much less popular and for the most part are no longer used. It is much better and more effective to take a single ingredient in the correct dose.

One occasional exception to this rule is Atrovent. Atrovent is a drug that blocks the cholinergic nerve pathway in the airways, thus reducing the tendency for them to go into spasm. It comes as a metered-dose inhaler. It has been approved by the FDA and has been found to be especially effective in relieving the cough of people with chronic bronchitis and emphysema. It is not used and is not indicated for use in the primary management of patients with asthma. However, many physicians have found that administration of Atrovent together with a beta agonist produces an additive and beneficial effect on the airways. Moreover, Atrovent has so little toxicity that in severe asthma trying it alongside a beta agonist is often warranted. The major side effect of Atrovent occurs if it inadvertently gets sprayed into the eye. Such spraying can induce severe eye damage in people who suffer from glaucoma.

A Special Word on Cough Medicines

Coughing is virtually always both a symptom and a cause of asthma. In other words, a cough, especially at night, may be the only sign that your asthma is active. However, coughing also makes your airways tighter and your asthma worse! Because of this, many people, including many doctors, recommend cough suppressants. Mild, over-the-counter cough suppressants are generally harmless as well as ineffective; prescription cough suppressants (including those containing codeine) are potentially dangerous for asthmatics. They may make you sleepy and reduce your breathing effort. They may also dry out your lung secretions, making mucus harder to raise. Thus, we rarely prescribe cough syrup with codeine. Our approach is to treat the reason for the cough, not the cough itself. Azmacort, the topical steroid discussed above, is especially helpful in relieving the nocturnal cough of asthma.

HOME AIR COMPRESSORS

For serious and chronic asthmatics, a home air compressor is a good way to administer both beta agonists and cromolyn. Delivery is extremely effective — much more so than metered aerosols. It works particularly well for small children, the severely ill, or the elderly.

To use these durable and dependable devices, a solution of the medication is placed in a small cup attached to a face mask or mouthpiece. When the machine is turned on the solution is *nebulized* — made into a fine mist, which is easily inhaled (Figure 18).

Where drugs need to be administered daily to small children or to severe asthmatics, these air compressors are strongly recommended. The cost, about $165, may seem like a drawback, but avoiding one emergency room visit will repay it. Most health plans — even government-subsidized insurance for the poor and underprivileged — will pay for a compressor if your doctor takes the time and trouble to demand it.

> When Terri was about 18 months old, during what appeared to be a routine cold with low-grade fever and runny nose, her parents noted that she was becoming uncomfortable and breathing rapidly. Her physician assured them that the wheezing was not serious and would likely disappear in a day or two. Some medication was prescribed, and the wheezing improved when the cold disappeared. Subsequently, every time Terri had a cold, wheezing set in. Some episodes were much more severe and frightening than others and required visits to hospital emergency rooms where epinephrine was injected. These always helped, although sometimes two or even three injections were needed.
>
> When Terri was three, she had a particularly severe bout of wheezing which did not respond to epinephrine injections. She had to be hospitalized and given oxygen, fluids, and intravenous drugs. Following discharge, the physician told the parents that she needed intensive preventive medicine to keep the wheezing under control. Accordingly, the parents purchased a DeVilbiss Pulmo-Aide air compressor. Thereafter, whenever Terri showed signs of respiratory infection, even before wheezing developed, her parents began to administer a solution of Bronkosol (a beta agonist) four to six times a day as directed by their physician. Although the wheezing continued during her cold, it was much more mild, and Terri required no more visits to the emergency room. As she grew older and her airways got larger, the seriousness of the wheezing decreased. At nine Terry still requires medication, but her parents feel that the turnaround in Terri's health came from the use of the home nebulizer.

Compressors come in several forms, including those that work on a battery pack or plug into the wall or a car's cigarette lighter. Most units are about the size of a shoe box or smaller. DURA Pharmaceuticals sells three portable units; one, the Tote-A-Neb 1500, has a rechargeable battery and can be carried and used virtually anywhere. The best buy, however, is the Pulmo-Travelmate by DeVilbiss. It is heavier than the Tote-A-Neb but is, in our opinion, more durable. (See Appendix H.)

OVER-THE-COUNTER ASTHMA MEDICATIONS

The availability of effective OTC medications for the relief of mild asthma symptoms has been one of the significant advances in medical treatment of the last two decades. Over-the-counter asthma medications work by relieving the bronchial constriction that results when the musculature surrounding the airways goes into spasm. The active ingredients are theophylline and/or beta agonists, which are delivered either in a hand-held nebulizer and sprayed directly into the airways or in the form of a tablet. Some people taking these drugs suffer the side effects of nausea, palpitations, and restlessness.

FIGURE 18   Use of a Home Air Compressor

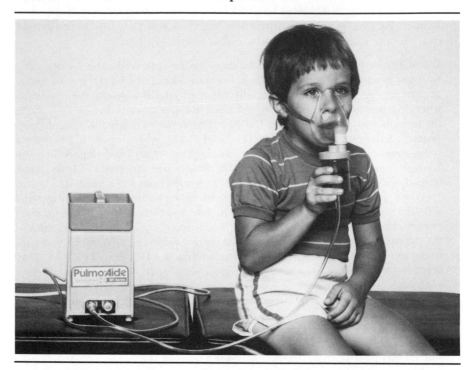

Primatene Mist is the most heavily advertised of the over-the-counter beta agonists. It can be extremely effective for the treatment of very mild symptoms and has been a boon to individuals who suffer from this mild form of asthma. However, it may produce undesirable side effects not associated with recently developed prescription medications like Maxair (Table 11). Patients may also develop tachyphylaxis, a tolerance to this type of medication which makes long term use less effective. We do not recommend routine use of Primatene Mist.

Table 15 lists the most important nonprescription bronchodilators, their form, and other active ingredients, and whether they are theophylline or beta agonist in their action. If you have mild, occasional bouts of asthma, you probably are able to control or ease your symptoms markedly by using one or another of this large array of nonprescription medications. If your asthma is bad enough for daily medication, then these OTC drugs are not for you. See your doctor for more effective medications.

Although OTC medications have made life more bearable for most asthmatics, they have had other, less agreeable consequences. Dramatic results have encouraged people to become overreliant on them and to ignore the other aspects of an effective, comprehensive program of asthma self-management — exercise, breathing improvement, careful avoidance of allergens, and so on. Second, these medications, especially if overused, carry side effects that can be extremely perilous. Moreover, many chronic asthmatics who require more effective medication do themselves a disservice by not taking the correct prescription medicine for their asthma.

TABLE 15 Over-the-Counter Bronchodilators*

| Drug Name and Form | Bronchodilator Agent | | |
	Theophylline	Beta Agonist	Additives
AsthmaNefrin solution with nebulizer 1 oz		epinephrine	chlorobutanol 0.5% (preservative)
Asthma-Meter Mist without nebulizer ½ oz		0.5% solution of epinephrine; 0.2 mg epinephrine per puff	ascorbic acid 0.1% (preservative) alcohol 34%
microNefrin 7.5 ml with nebulizer		2.25% epinephrine	sodium chloride, sodium bisulfite, potassium metabisulfite, potassium metabisulfite 0.074 mg/7.5 ml
Primatene Mist ½ oz without nebulizer		0.05% solution of epinephrine; 0.2 mg epinephrine per puff	ascorbic acid (preservative); alcohol 34%
Bronkaid Mist with nebulizer ½ oz		0.5% solution of epinephrine; 0.2 mg epinephrine per puff	ascorbic acid (preservative); alcohol 34%
Bronkaid tablets	theophylline 100 mg/tablet	ephedrine 24 mg/tablet	guanifesin 100 mg/tablet
Primatene M tablets	theophylline 130 mg/tablet	ephedrine 24 mg/tablet	M-pyrilamine maleate 16 mg/tablet
Primatene P tablets	theophylline 130 mg/tablet	ephedrine 24 mg/tablet	P-phenobarbital 8 mg/tablet
Tedral tablets	theophylline 118 mg/tablet	ephedrine 24 mg/tablet	phenobarbital 8 mg/tablet
Amodrine tablets	aminophylline 100 mg/tablet	ephedrine 25 mg/tablet	phenobarbital 8 mg/tablet
Asma-Lief tablets	theophylline 130 mg/tablet	ephedrine 24 mg/tablet	phenobarbital 8 mg/tablet
AsthmaHaler oral inhalant		epinephrine 7 mg/ml	
Breatheasy oral inhalant (Pascal)		epinephrine	benzyl alcohol 1%
Bronitin tablets	theophylline 130 mg/tablet	ephedrine 24 mg/tablet	guanifesin 100 mg/tablet pyrilamine maleate 16 mg/tablet
Vaponefrin solution		2.25% epinephrine	chlorobutanol 0.5%
Phedral tablets	theophylline 130 mg/tablet	ephedrine 24 mg/tablet	phenobarbital 8.1 mg/tablet
Thalfed tablets	theophylline 120 mg/tablet	ephedrine 25 mg/tablet	phenobarbital 8 mg/tablet
Azura Aid tablets	theophylline 118 mg/tablet	ephedrine 24 mg/tablet	phenobarbital 8 mg/tablet
Tedrigen tablets	theophylline 125 mg/tablet	ephedrine/TCI 25 mg/tablet	phenobarbital 8 mg/tablet
Bronchotabs	theophylline 100 mg/tablet	ephedrine sulfate 24 mg/tablet	guanifesin 100 mg phenobarbital 8 mg

*These drugs can cause nausea, vomiting, palpitations, or restlessness in some people.

16 Allergy Shots and Asthma Treatment

HOW DO ALLERGY SHOTS WORK?

Desensitization, or the reduction in your allergic state, is achieved by administering a series of increasingly more potent shots of the allergen that is causing your symptoms. It is an accepted and commonplace method of treating certain allergies. This desensitization process has an uneven record of success in asthma, in contrast to that for hay fever. For hay fever sufferers, where the allergen is definitely known and where the symptoms are not easily controlled by other means, desensitization usually works and represents a real blessing. The use of allergy shots to manage asthma is not as likely to succeed.

Desensitization rests on a homeopathic principle whose roots go back to the very beginnings of medicine. It relies on the discovery that very minute amounts of substances, which in larger quantities cause severe reactions, can be tolerated by the body. These minuscule doses can systematically be made more potent by very small degrees so that, after a period of time, the individual can tolerate quantities of the substance that would earlier have caused serious or even fatal illness. For allergy sufferers, this gradual process of desensitization brings the threshold of reaction up to the point where the concentration of allergen occurring naturally in the environment no longer produces the allergic symptoms.

THE ROLE OF ALLERGY SHOTS IN ASTHMA TREATMENT

A series of allergy shots may be useful if it is definitely established that your asthma is a reaction to an allergen. Allergy shots ought to be administered for asthma *only* if strict and careful avoidance strategies have not worked and if medications have proven ineffective. Allergy shots or immunotherapy should rarely be used as the *sole* treatment of asthma.

Allergy shots have been used for years in attempts to reduce allergic reactions. The basic method of making allergenic extracts has improved very little during the last 50 years, although the means to standardize and control manufacturing, testing, and storage do exist. The standard practice has been to soak an allergen such as grass pollen in a solution containing saline (salt) or in some other buffered solution to leach out the allergen. Then the allergen is sterilized by filtration. Obviously, there are several conditions one hopes (but cannot be sure) are being met. The material being injected should be free of extraneous material; it should be potent, stable, and efficacious.

Unfortunately, in only a handful of instances are there standard potencies for allergy shots, and almost never is the final product tested to determine its strength or even its composition. Recently there have been efforts to standardize the potency of allergenic extracts in the form of protein nitrogen units (PNU), which describe the concentration of allergen in a given preparation. This has been successful with such allergens as insect venoms in which the compound responsible for the allergic response has been isolated. However, in the case of molds this level of standardization has not been achieved. At present, allergy is the only field of medicine to employ injectable substances that are not required to have guaranteed potency or authoritative dosage recommendations based on intensive studies.

Some extracts are prepared crudely, while others are carefully made under acceptably controlled conditions. At one extreme there is house dust. A large number of patients with allergy and asthma are allergic to house dust, and it is found everywhere. However, it is very difficult to determine what is in house dust. It contains every sort of particulate matter as well as dust mites and bodies of other insects. Its basic biochemical composition varies enormously from house to house. There is persuasive evidence that the triggering agent in house dust may be the excreta of the house dust mite.

In some cases allergen manufacturers get the house dust they use in preparing their extracts from the contents of vacuum cleaner bags. In other instances, they use the dust found on mattress covers. It is not surprising, therefore, that tremendous variation exists from batch to batch and company to company with respect to house dust allergen potency and efficacy.

At the other extreme is the extract prepared to treat allergy to bee stings. Allergy to honeybees and other stinging insects like wasps, hornets, yellow jackets, and fire ants is found often in individuals who reside in the country, in beekeepers, and in people who work outdoors. For many years individuals allergic to bee stings were treated (desensitized) by receiving injections of extracts made from the ground-up bodies of bees. This was thought to be a highly effective procedure until about a decade ago when some imaginative studies demonstrated that these whole-body extracts of bees were not working at all. The experiments proved conclusively that the allergen from a bee sting is the venom itself. They went on to show that if you injected only the venom into susceptible individuals a blocking antibody would be produced by that person. Indeed, it has been definitely shown that bee venom shots ultimately eliminate allergic reactions to bee stings in most people. As a result of this discovery, rigorous procedures have been developed for producing venom extracts of known and controlled potency.

The Food and Drug Administration has only recently begun to address these critical issues. The next several years should see major new pioneering efforts to develop allergens that meet approved criteria. Our ability to clone biological molecules will play a significant role in preparing allergenic extracts that are pure and have accurate concentrations.

Who Should Receive Allergy Shots?

The only individuals who should receive allergy shots for asthma are those who have extrinsic or IgE-mediated disease as revealed by skin tests or a clear unequivocal history. Other asthmatics do not need to be given allergy shots. Accordingly, very small children who have asthma brought on by virus infections should not receive allergy shots nor should individuals whose skin tests are negative. Generally we do not recommend allergy skin testing for children under four. In most cases a physician can tell by your history whether allergy shots are indicated or not. Just because you have positive tests does not necessarily mean that you would benefit from shots, however.

Evan has had eczema, hay fever, and asthma all of his life. His eczema is a problem 12 months a year and is especially troublesome in hot weather. It is usually mild to moderate but has been adequately controlled through use of cortisone creams and avoidance of caustic agents. Evan's hay fever is generally similar to his asthma in that it is particularly bad in the spring and the fall when things pollinate. He is also very allergic to dust.

Evan's allergist suspected that Evan would be allergic to most pollens as well as to house dust, but she wanted to confirm her hunch. She did the skin tests, and the tests for pollens and dusts turned out positive. Evan was elated because he thought that, because he had a positive skin test, his allergies and especially his asthma might be relieved with allergy shots.

His allergist told him that she was reluctant to give him allergy shots because of his eczema, believing that the shots might make his eczema worse. She preferred to treat Evan with a more vigorous program of medications in the spring and fall to suppress the hay fever and the asthma symptoms.

Evan decided it was time to see another allergist. He sought out a physician who advertised that he treated allergies by nutritional and "preventive medicine" means and advocated the use of a whole variety of "ecological" procedures, including special testing known as cytotoxic testing.

This new physician said that Evan should receive allergy shots and Evan readily agreed. He began a program of twice-a-week injections. After about three months his hay fever and his asthma had not improved. Moreover, his eczema was becoming much more severe and stubborn. It was not responding as well as it had before and was causing a great deal more itching. Evan conceded the first allergist had been right and he discontinued the shots.

Although some allergists occasionally treat people who have hay fever, asthma, and eczema with allergy shots, we believe that unless there is an overriding reason — as in the case of someone who is just not responding to other drugs — allergy shots should not be used in people with eczema.

Some asthma patients with positive skin tests may have a gratifying response.

Allen first developed asthma at age 12. His wheezing persisted 12 months a year and was always made worse by smoke, polluted air, and exercise. His asthma was particularly bad during the spring and for a short period during the fall. Thus, although he had asthma year round, there was clearly a seasonal exacerbation of his problem. He was referred to an allergist who did a panel of skin tests. The skin tests were found to be positive for trees, grasses, weeds, and dust. The allergist began a program of weekly hyposensitization shots for Allen. After a period of about six months Allen was gratified to notice that his asthma for most of the year was much the same but during spring and fall the rise or the exacerbation that he normally would see was blunted and his asthma was considerably easier to manage.

How Are Allergy Shots Done?

The first step in preparing an immunization schedule for your allergy shots, sometimes called a vaccine, is to find out what you are allergic to by giving tests. After the tests are completed and the offender pinned down, a dilute mixture of the allergens you are sensitive to is prepared. The first injection will be a very weak solution — possibly one part vaccine to one million parts saline solution. Thereafter, once or twice a week you will receive an injection of allergen in your arm. Following each injection you must stay in the doctor's office for 30 minutes in case a systemic reaction develops. Before you leave your arm is inspected to see whether or not there has been a local reaction to the shot. If you develop any discomfort at all following the shots you are immediately seen by a physician.

Assuming that you show no local or systemic reactions, the strength of the dose of allergen increases each time. If things go well a dose strength of l part allergen to 100 parts vehicle is eventually reached and maintained.

Some physicians take all the allergens you are sensitive to and mix them in one vial, while others prefer to administer separate shots. Thus you may have one shot or separate shots for trees, grass, house dust, and so on, depending on your allergist's experience and your own degree of sensitivity.

We do not advocate testing or immunizing for food allergy in asthmatics. Skin testing for asthma resulting from food allergies is rarely useful and may even provoke life-threatening reactions (see Chapter 5).

How Long Should Allergy Shots Be Continued?

Allergy shots usually go on for a period of approximately six months to one year. If, after that time, your allergies do not seem to be better under control (fewer and/or less severe episodes), discontinue the shots. On the other hand, should you have an affirmative response, continue them for another year or two until, depending on your response and the nature of your allergies, their frequency will be decreased. For example, at that point, instead of having a shot once a week, you may have a shot every other week or even once a month. This is an individual decision and one that should be made in consultation with your doctor.

The Dangers of Allergy Shots

Allergy shots are potent extracts of the material that you are allergic to. Since they are being injected directly into your body, they have the potential for inducing an acute anaphylactic reaction, a form of shock which may result in death. In fact, the *single most common cause of anaphylaxis is injection of allergy extracts*. It is for this reson that they should always be done under a doctor's supervision and emergency equipment to treat anaphylaxis should be *immediately* available. Those having allergy shots should let their doctors know of any local reactions and any systemic complaints they may provoke. Systemic complains may include wheezing, shortness of breath, swelling of the face or throat, and hives. If these occur, then the doctor will probably reduce the strength of the allergy shot for several weeks. If you are receiving a dose at 1:1000 dilution and begin to experience large local reactions, you should have your dose cut back to a dilution of perhaps 1:10,000 and maintained at that level for a time. Later, as the dose is increased, you should have developed some immunity, which will prevent these reactions. There are many people who are so sensitive that they cannot tolerate large doses of allergy extracts. Others are so sensitive to specific agents that they must omit them from their treatment vial or else have them administered singly in extremely dilute solution.

Allergy Shots to Counteract Sensitivity of Pets

One of the more melancholy chores of an allergist entails advising an asthmatic's family to remove the family dog or cat. All too often this advice is rejected, or else the family rationalizes that the pet is an outdoor animal. Allergies to animals can be serious. The pets may not produce obvious symptoms, but they may have enough impact to push you over the edge when you are wheezing from other causes. Many people found to be allergic to their pets insist on having allergy shots to desensitize them to the animals. Although such shots are available, we discourage them. First, the small amount of evidence available suggests that such shots often fail to work. Second, the extracts from animals may make your allergies get worse. Third, the extracts are prepared from skin cells from animals, and these skin cells may contain viruses that can trigger infections or diseases.

Only in the cases of individuals who *must* be exposed to animals do we administer allergy shots for animal dander. By far the largest group are veterinarians who have allergies to pets. Families who insist on allergy injections in preference to giving up their pets are sometimes accommodated, but the procedure is risky, expensive, prolonged, and frequently ineffectual.

BACTERIAL VACCINES

For a number of years it was popular to treat recurrent infections and asthma and sinusitis by administering bacterial or autologous vaccines. In this process a culture containing bacteria from the individual's throat or sinus discharge is cultivated. The bacteria are then heat killed and vaccines prepared. In other cases, commercially prepared vaccines containing extracts of the common bacteria that infect people were available. Despite the theoretical possibility that this procedure ought to work, it has never been shown to be effective. In some cases, toxic responses have followed administration of bacterial vaccines. Bacterial vaccines are no longer recommended, and we strongly discourage their clinical use.

GAMMA GLOBULIN

Gamma globulin is an important substance in the working of our immune systems. Injections of gamma globulin are sometimes given to people with impaired immune systems whose bodies cannot produce it themselves. Recently there has been research interest in administering such injections to people with asthma. We believe that gamma globulin should be given only to patients with very severe symptoms that do not respond to conventional drugs. Besides being very expensive, gamma globulin carries the risk of provoking a serious allergic reaction.

The Treatment
of Acute Asthma

In a severe asthma attack there is considerable tightness in the chest. Sometimes it almost feels as if there were an iron band around it. Breathing becomes rapid, shallow, and difficult, and even the slightest exertion — like a spell of coughing, for example — will leave you spent and panting. Wheezing will be loud enough to be heard by another person halfway across a fairly large room, and there will be an overabundance of thick, clinging, yellow-tinged mucus, which will be extremely difficult to raise. If these conditions develop, do the following:

1. Try and determine what, if anything, triggered the reaction. For example, was it an infection, exposure to an allergen, a recent period of exercise, or something you cannot single out?
2. Make sure you are taking the recommended doses of medication. If you are told to increase your medication during a bout of asthma, do so at once.
3. Increase your fluid intake. Rapid, shallow breathing causes a drastic loss of body fluid, which must be replaced. An adequate supply of liquids is essential to keep mucus thin.
4. Try and raise your mucus and prevent clogging of mucus in your airways. (See Chapter 14.)
5. Avoid any other medication that may make your asthma worse. In particular, *avoid aspirin and any sedatives.*
6. Take your temperature and determine if you have a fever.
7. Monitor your respiration rate or that of your child. Normal adults breathe at the rate of 16 – 20 breaths per minute; children breathe at a rate of 20 – 25 breaths per minute. Infants take between 30 and 40 breaths per minute. If you or your child's respiratory rate becomes

consistently elevated, it should be noted and you should alert your physician.

One of the more embarrassing things for asthmatics is trying to control their cough and wheezing in public areas. If you begin to have symptoms and need to use your metered aerosol, do not hesitate. It is far less embarrassing to you in the long run.

Diane, a college student, has moderate chronic asthma. During class she felt her chest tighten up and her wheezing begin. This came as no surprise. She hadn't felt all that well that day and had been wheezing the night before. The class had 35 minutes to go. She could hear herself wheezing and thought that everyone around her heard her too. She knew she ought to reach for her inhaler but decided to try to wait until the end of the hour. With about 10 minutes to go she couldn't hold out any longer and went into a severe episode of coughing and choking. The professor and her classmates came to her aid, but eventually she had to be taken to the emergency room of the Student Health Center. When asked about it later, Diane said she hadn't used her medication because she was too embarrassed to get up and walk out in the middle of the lecture and too self-conscious to use the inhaler right there at her seat. She said that she didn't want to draw attention to herself.

WHEN TO CALL A DOCTOR

If any of the following conditions turn up during the course of an asthma attack, consult your doctor as soon as possible.

- Fever
- Vomiting and abdominal pain
- Persistent rapid respiratory rate that does not return to normal
- Wheezing and shortness of breath that does not respond to medications

Fever may indicate the presence of infection and other illnesses, which can drastically complicate ordinary asthmatic episodes. Sometimes mucus ends up by being swallowed into the stomach, causing vomiting, particularly in children. Some of the medications used to treat asthma, such as theophyllines, lead to gastric irritation and vomiting. In fact, one problem in children is that parents administer larger-than-prescribed doses of theophylline because the symptoms do not abate. Then children become sick from the overdosage and vomit. The chronic cough and the air hunger that asthmatics have may cause stomach bloating, which can also lead to abdominal pain and vomiting.

Vomiting can be a very serious complication for asthmatics. If you vomit you lose body fluids and become dehydrated. Dehydration in turn makes mucus thicker and reduces air flow. Also, vomiting prevents you from being able to keep your medication down. If any of this occurs, it is important that you see your physician immediately! Likewise, if your respiratory rate remains persistently above normal, or if usually effective medications do not improve wheezing or breathing, call your doctor.

A SPECIAL WARNING ABOUT SEDATIVES

It is uncommon for anyone to die of asthma. However, one of the most common things found in people who *do* die from it is the fact that they had been taking sedative agents or tranquilizers. If you have an acute asthma attack you must keep your respiratory drive as strong as possible. It is also important that you possess all of your mental function. If you take a sedative you become sleepy and your respiratory muscles get sluggish. The result is drifting off, a further decline in respiratory function, unconsciousness, and death from lack of oxygen. *Under no circumstance should anybody with asthma ever take a sedative.*

Jill is eight years of age and has had asthma for the past four years. She becomes terribly anxious whenever she begins to wheeze. Her mother has often felt that her anxiety and the fact that Jill is often hyperactive anyway caused the asthma in the first place. She consulted her pediatrician, who told her that he did not want to give Jill any tranquilizers for asthma. He explained that they can make asthma worse. However, Jill's mother decided she would give her some of her own tranquilizers. She gave Jill 2 mg of Valium about three times a day. Jill's hyperactivity actually seemed to get better for a few days. However, Jill was sleepy much of the time.

About two weeks later Jill developed a cold; it began to settle in her chest and made her wheezing worse. Jill's mother decided to double the dose of Valium. Although Jill had been wheezing for the past four years, she never required hospitalization. However, during this episode, Jill just couldn't seem to get enough air; she got sleepy and her respiration became shallow. Her mother panicked and rushed her to the emergency room. Jill was examined and found to be in *status asthmaticus* (the most severe form of asthma), with severe obstruction. The doctor determined that Jill's respiratory reserve was insufficient, and he hospitalized her and performed an intubation to place her on an artificial respirator. Jill's pediatrician could not understand what precipitated this severe episode. Jill's mother finally admitted she had been giving her daughter tranquilizers.

NIGHTTIME ASTHMA

For many asthmatics the nighttime period is the worst. The reason for this is unknown. At bedtime they feel well, take their medicine, and go to sleep. Then in the dark hours of the early morning they wake up wheezing. Many reasons have been advanced to account for this: nighttime accumulation of mucus in the lungs; the fact that the body has different rhythms in the daytime versus the nighttime. It may arise from dust being released in the air vents during the night, or it may have to do with other allergens present in the room, such as dust mites in the bed or bedding.

Nighttime asthma is best prevented by taking one of the long-acting theophyllines or by using cromolyn sodium regularly. If your child is affected and begins wheezing in the middle of the night, you may have to wake him or her up and administer an inhaler (beta agonists). This is far better than having the child continue to wheeze and cough throughout the night, only to awaken the next morning with tight, constricted, mucus-jammed airways.

HOSPITALIZATION FOR AN ASTHMATIC EMERGENCY

Admission for acute severe asthma is among the most frequent causes of hospitalization in any community. There is nothing more dramatic and frightening than the acute shortness of breath seen in a wheezing individual. The inability to get enough air arouses tremendous feelings of fear in observers and victims, even though it usually looks worse than it actually is.

When you are being evaluated in an emergency, the doctors or attendants will do a number of things. First, they will assess the severity of your reactions so that they may provide the acute care you need. Acute care may entail administering oxygen, fluids, and medication. To decide what you need quickly, emergency room personnel may appear brusque, impersonal, and dispassionate. This does not mean they are uncaring. On the other hand, if the staff ask you to fill out forms or supply information while you can't breathe, complain. You know how you feel and, if you need to see a doctor immediately, on the spot, *demand it!* An asthmatic episode serious enough to have you at the emergency room requires special, prompt attention.

If you are transporting someone to the hospital, move them quickly but without endangering yourself and others. Don't risk an automobile accident. Stay cool and calm. If transportation is not available or symptoms are very severe, dial 911. The fire department and rescue squad always carry oxygen and will bring you directly to the closest available hospital.

Emergency Room Procedures

Entering the emergency room in the throes of a severe asthmatic reaction sets off a series of events. First, you will be taken to a station and seated. If necessary, oxygen will be administered. Then someone will take your vital signs — your heart rate, blood pressure, respiratory rate, and, sometimes, your temperature. Next, a physician or nurse practitioner will probably listen to your lungs. At this stage the first direct countermeasures will be taken.

A child having a severe asthmatic attack will receive either an injection of Adrenalin (epinephrine) or an aerosol treatment, whichever can be given more quickly. More physicians now prefer aerosolized bronchodilators such as Alupent and Ventolin because of their relative safety and limited side effects. However, an injection of Adrenalin almost always produces dramatically rapid improvement — usually within a matter of seconds. One shot may be all that is required, but if it produces only temporary relief, a second and even a third injection may be necessary.

Only a limited number of Adrenalin shots can be given, because they can be harmful and dangerous. Adrenalin or epinephrine can cause the heart to race alarmingly and may produce feelings of nausea. Some individuals develop pounding headaches or even migraine after receiving Adrenalin. However, one shot usually works; Adrenalin is an effective and time-honored method of treating the symptoms of acute asthmatic reactions.

There is also a special form of epinephrine called susphrine. This is actually epinephrine suspended in an oil base. It permits a delayed and sustained release of the drug and thus extends the duration of the effect of epinephrine. Usually the effect of an epinephrine shot lasts 20 minutes; susphrine extends the action to four to six hours. However, we do *not* recommend its use, because in episodes of acute asthma we prefer to know exactly what the response is to a specific dose of medication. Susphrine, because of its prolonged and somewhat unpredictable effects, makes this sort of strategy impossible to follow.

Adrenalin shots are no longer given to older children and adults. The reason for this is that there are now drugs in the Adrenalin family that can be given by aerosol. These drugs are generally administered as a fine mist using a nebulizer. The mist is inhaled and, like Adrenalin shots, the nebulized drug works within minutes, producing a dramatic remission of symptoms.

If the injection of Adrenalin or the inhalation therapy does not produce improvement, other steps will be initiated. At this point the child or adult is usually admitted to the hospital and intravenous drugs and fluids given. The purpose of the intravenous tube is to supply fluids to fight off the dehydration, often a companion of asthma. The reason for this is simple. The rapid, shallow breathing that is a part of asthma causes a serious loss of body fluids especially important in the body's struggle against asthma.

The intravenous line may also be used to carry other asthma-fighting drugs. Usually the drug administered at this point (and assuming a clear diagnosis of asthma) will be theophylline, the same drug prescribed for oral use for chronic asthmatics. When administered intravenously, a large load can be introduced into the body in a short time and a therapeutically effective level of the medicine established quickly and maintained.

Once the acute attack is controlled or stabilized, additional tests may be ordered. These can include a chest X ray as well as a test to determine the amount of oxygen in the blood. The chest X ray shows whether there are any abnormalities within the lung other than the effects of asthma itself. Here the physician looks for underlying pneumonia or a collapsed airway, or some defect in air movement through the lung, which has permitted air to leak out into the chest wall or into the lung cavity itself; the latter is called a pneumothorax. These conditions all require special immediate treatment.

The arterial blood gas test capitalizes on the knowledge that the arteries carry oxygen directly from the lungs. By taking some blood from an artery, the laboratory is able to tell the physician how much oxygen is dissolved in the blood. It gives a precise measure of the severity of the asthma, and it is also an excellent way to monitor the effectiveness of the therapy being given. In most cases it is necessary to do the arterial puncture, or "stick," only once. The improvement that occurs with treatment is usually so obvious that further arterial punctures are not necessary. In the few instances where repeated sticks are necessary, there will be some local discomfort, but the test is only a bit more painful than any other routine blood test. The major complication of the arterial stick is the risk of bleeding. Your doctor should hold pressure over the stick site for several minutes following the test. Then a pressure bandage is applied. (As with any blood test, if the person doing it is having trouble finding the artery, ask for an "expert" to help. You are probably miserable enough without having a novice practice on you. Asking for an anesthesiologist to help with arterial sticks is sometimes a good idea. These specialists have the most experience in drawing blood.)

There is a new method of measuring oxygen content in the blood that does not require a needle stick, called pulse oximetry. This method does not provide as much useful data as an arterial blood gas test, but it is much less painful and therefore often preferable.

It may also be necessary, in the hospital, to get help from an inhalation therapist. These specialists will administer the beta agonists like the Alupent you take as a hand-held, metered aerosol. The inhalation therapist will deliver it through the special ventilating equipment used in the emergency room. These machines provide good aerosolized medication.

In addition, patients admitted to the hospital are almost always given high doses of intravenous steroids or cortisone. This is probably the single best drug available to break off their attack. However, it requires several hours to work and then must be continued for several days before the attack is considered completely gone. Even then, there may be some residual wheezing, and certainly, if pulmonary function testing is done, some abnormalities can be seen. Probably the biggest mistake in the treatment of severe asthma is not to give enough steroids or to stop them too soon. Prolonged use of steroids is associated with serious side effects, but you should take them as long as your doctor prescribes them. If you stop too early, the acute asthma will rebound, often worse than the initial episode. When this happens, another hospital visit is required, and the ordeal of going through all of these steps is repeated. Generally, hospitalization for acute asthma lasts no longer than three or four days.

THE USE OF A RESPIRATOR OR VENTILATOR

Asthmatics rarely need to be put on a respirator, but a respirator may be called into use when one becomes exhausted and unable to breathe independently. It may also be called in when the results of the physical exam, the pulmonary function tests, and the blood gas analysis are so ominous that the physician fears a sudden respiratory or even heart collapse. In that case, the doctor may elect to put you on a ventilator before the emergency happens, rather than try an emergency intubation during a cardiac or respiratory arrest. Realistically, only your physician will know what signs to look for and can decide on this drastic step. Cyanosis, a dark blue or purplish coloration of the skin due to lack of oxygen, is one of the signs physicians frequently encounter and are especially concerned about. It is a *late* sign, which denotes a severe lack of oxygen and truly indicates an emergency.

If your physician elects to intubate you, he or she usually calls in an anesthesiologist and places you in intensive care. At that time you will receive some medication to make you sleepy and thus less likely to feel the trauma of having a tracheostomy or air tube inserted and being hooked up to a machine. While most people absolutely dread the thought of having a tube down their throat, virtually all admit after it is done that it was not nearly as bad as they imagined it would be.

Roger has been on a camping trip in the Sierra Mountains for the past week. Although he has had asthma for many years, he finds that it no longer troubles him and he lives a full, active, and vigorous life. Unfortunately, he was not used to climbing, and although his body was in good shape for ordinary athletic activities he found that climbing, with its reduced level of oxygen and the extreme exertion, was too much for him. At about 9500 feet he collapsed. He developed an acute shortness of breath and turned blue. His companion had no means to contact help other than to leave Roger on the mountainside and descend to the base camp for assistance. It was several hours before a relief team got to Roger. By that time he was unconscious and unarousable. He was brought to a local hospital where treatment of his acute asthma, as well as the acute pulmonary edema that he developed from climbing, was begun. The physicians wanted permission from Roger to intubate him. By this time Roger was conscious but not especially coherent. He visualized the intubation process as reducing him to a vegetable status for the rest of his life and balked, but his terrible shortness of breath and desperate struggle to breathe finally led him to give grudging permission. Although the process was uncomfortable for Roger, he found out within a few hours that he tolerated it quite well. Moreover, it made his body relax and it released him from the need to breathe as hard and as deep as he could because the machine did most of the work. Roger went home four days later as fit as when he began his camping trip.

Whatever else may be said about hospitalization, it provides an excellent opportunity, after the acute problem is resolved, to find out why it happened. This is also the time to review the steps of prevention. Was this another instance of poorly controlled asthma that could have been prevented? What lessons are there? In addition, look back over your own care. Check the services and care provided by your physician. Was your medication and treatment schedule optimal? Did you know as much as you should have when you entered the hospital? Were you inadvertently exposed to an allergen which precipitated your attack? Go over the medicines on discharge to make sure that you understand the instructions. Be sure to take the drugs recommended at the intervals and in the amounts prescribed.

CAN ASTHMA KILL?

Deaths do result from asthma. In fact, in spite of our increased knowledge about asthma, the mortality rate for asthma has increased over the past 15 years. Fortunately, most patients with asthma, particularly adults, never require hospital admission for this disease, so the overall death rate from asthma is extremely low. Some of the reasons why people do die from their asthma include the following:

1. *They are given sedatives.*
The panic that occurs from shortness of breath makes asthmatics extremely agitated. Accordingly, some may take or be given tranquilizing agents that have been either prescribed for other family members or sometimes incorrectly prescribed for themselves. Sedatives or tranquilizers (Librium, Valium) should *never* be used by asthmatics.

2. *They overmedicate, especially with beta agonists or theophyllines.*
Often asthmatics in the throes of an attack think that if they increase the dose of the medicine they could better control their symptoms. To some extent this is true, but only within limits; continuing to increase medication without an obvious response is foolhardy. All it does is increase the toxicity of these drugs. Some of this toxicity may be manifested in the heart and may produce heart irregularities. Instead of significantly increasing your dose, go to the emergency room or see your doctor immediately.

3. *They undermedicate, which can lead to a sudden, lethal attack or episode.*
Know and be sure of the correct doses of your medication and take them faithfully. Do not decide you can undertreat yourself and try and get away with the least amount of drug possible.

4. *They expose themselves to allergens more frequently because they can control their symptoms with medications.*
Medicines that relieve aggravating symptoms don't remove the allergy itself. Increased exposure to substances that incite asthma can lead to more attacks of greater severity.

18 Summer Camps and Other Special Treatment and Care Programs

Over the years a number of different programs have been developed whose common objective is to provide comprehensive and aggressive treatment of asthma, coupled with intensive, broadly based education about the disease and training in its self-management. Primarily aimed at providing help to children with moderate to severe or intractable asthma, these programs vary greatly in focus, duration, and intensity of therapeutic intervention. There are three different sorts of programs:

1. Summer camps
2. Community-based programs for training or outpatient treatment
3. Long-term residential care facilities

SUMMER CAMPS

Summer camps for asthmatic children began in the late 1950s when a group of young physicians rejected the then prevailing notion of what constituted appropriate treatment for asthmatic children. These rebels contended (correctly) that asthmatics did not need to lead an isolated, sedentary existence and that, with proper care, training, and supervision they could participate in and enjoy many activities previously denied them. This led to the establishment of summer camps especially designed for moderately to severely asthmatic children. These camps offered ongoing medical supervision and a program of activities aimed at accomplishing two goals. First, they tried to provide experiences, enjoyable for their own sake, that these children had been denied in the past. Second, the intent was to help the campers (and, in some instances, their parents) develop a knowledge of and control over all aspects of the disease and its treatment — to aid the children in attaining the ability to manage and control their symptoms more effectively. The educational programs vary widely from camp to camp, from a basic transmission of information to a tightly organized self-management training program that may even consider the psychosocial issues that so often complicate the disease.

167
SUMMER CAMPS
AND OTHER
SPECIAL
TREATMENT AND
CARE PROGRAMS

This once daring and hotly debated move has proved to be extremely successful. Summer asthma camps with names like Camp Superkids, Camp Wheeze, and Camp Huff 'n Puff have sprung up throughout the country. These are generally sponsored and financially supported by local lung associations or chapters of the Asthma and Allergy Foundation of America, but they have attracted a wide range of other backers: thoracic, pediatric, and allergic societies; religious groups, Children's Aid; medical societies; and private organizations all fund and staff these camps.

To locate the nearest asthma camp, call the American Lung Association for information and referrals. The phone number will be in your local white pages. The *Asthma Resources Directory* (see Appendix H) includes a list of camps. Unfortunately, not all localities have this valuable resource for children. The number of applicants to any camp may exceed the spaces available, so preference is usually given to children with moderate to severe symptoms who have had no prior camping experience. A doctor's statement is invariably required, and the application asks for a complete history of the child's episodes and an enumeration of causes and special dietary, medication, and other needs.

The camps are often staffed by former campers, themselves asthmatics, who understand — and respond sensitively to — the needs, problems, and anxieties of the children, some of whom are away from home for the first time and understandably frightened at the prospect. Medical needs, including adherence to medication schedules and management of any medical emergencies, are attended to by a resident medical staff (doctors and nurses), often volunteers from local pediatric or allergy societies. Dietary restrictions are noted and provided for, and the possibility of individuals violating their food restrictions is kept to a minimum.

In the last few years there have been two interesting developments. One of them is the establishment of camps where all sorts of infirmities are welcomed and managed together. In these camps it is not uncommon to have children who suffer from any one of a score or more of disabling conditions — asthma, cystic fibrosis, sickle cell anemia, muscular dystrophy, spinal cord injuries, diabetes, cerebral palsy — to be taken at the same time. A second development is "mainstreaming" the asthmatics, that is, having them attend camp with "regular" children. Whereas the asthmatic camper still has his or her special needs looked after, and some program elements continue to be directed specifically at managing the disease, the aim here is to have asthmatic and well children encounter and learn from one another. The anecdotal reports indicate that this sort of experience is especially valuable for asthmatic and nonasthmatic children alike. (See also Chapter 19 for considerations when attending regular summer camp for children with mild or seasonal asthma.)

Although the curriculum varies from one camp to another, most camps offer a course of instruction in the disease, provide skill training in use of medications, use an ingenious collection of breathing exercises (for example, "Puff Hockey," where teams arranged on sides of a Ping-Pong table try to blow a Ping-Pong ball into a goal), and run according to a settled routine that carries over to the home situation. In some instances the parents are encouraged to participate as well. Follow-up indicates that much of the information is retained for a significant period after camp and that campers show a drop in number of ill days, days absent from school, and emergency room visits in the year following camp.

Added to these benefits for the children is one for the parents. It is a period, however short, during which they are spared the ever-present burden of caring for their asthmatic child. To have the load lifted, even for a brief time, and placed on competent, knowledgeable shoulders is a rare gift.

Your decision whether to send your asthmatic child to a special camp should be based on your own knowledge of your child's condition, your physician's recommendation, and a consideration of the facilities offered by the camp itself. The campers have problems similar to your child's, and the staff know how to manage them. If they cannot handle your child's problem they will be the first to let you know. (In most instances, a medical panel evaluates each application and decides whether the camp facilities are sufficient for any special problems that your child may present.) Camp is an exceedingly worthwhile experience for most moderate to severe asthmatic children, and we strongly recommend that you seriously consider having your child participate. The potential benefits to you and the youngster far outweigh the risk.

COMMUNITY-BASED PROGRAMS FOR TRAINING OR OUTPATIENT TREATMENT

It is fair to say that most asthmatic symptoms, with appropriate treatment, can be either prevented or quickly controlled. That this ideal often does not occur in practice has more to do with breakdowns in communication between physician, parent, and asthmatic than deficiencies in available medical measures. Misunderstanding, failure to comprehend or adhere to procedures, inappropriate or unnecessarily heroic measures in response to crisis, and ineffectual, panic-fueled reactions growing out of feelings of helplessness, all conspire to make asthma more of a problem than it needs to be. Recognition of this side of the asthma problem has led to the establishment of a number of different kinds of community-based programs aimed at helping asthmatics and their parents know more about asthma and develop skill in the management of its symptoms. These self-management programs are offered by hospitals, schools, and community groups.

169
SUMMER CAMPS
AND OTHER
SPECIAL
TREATMENT AND
CARE PROGRAMS

Hospitals

There are a number of major allergy centers and clinics at hospitals throughout the country, which your health insurer should be able to tell you about. In addition to providing up-to-the-minute treatment and care, many of these institutions offer outpatient programs designed to educate asthmatics in the effective management of asthmatic symptoms. The programs vary from place to place. Most of them have the participants come together once weekly for an hour or two over a period of from four to eight weeks. The programs ordinarily include educational sessions that entail distribution and study of written materials, family and peer group support sessions, and behavior training experiences. They may also provide recreation, a telephone hot line during (and after) the course of instruction, and long-term follow-up. Parents are expected to accompany their children; sessions may be either separate or joint, depending on the program.

These programs aim to increase understanding, to teach self-management skills and techniques, to cut down frequency and severity of attacks (including reducing the frequency of emergency room visits), and to reduce school absenteeism. Evaluations of the programs indicate that most of the objectives are achieved with some degree of success.

While these hospital-based programs are not yet widespread, they seem to be a valuable adjunct to routine medical care. It would be worthwhile to locate one in your area.

Schools

The school is an obvious place to offer primarily educational programs aimed at asthmatic children. Considering the number of schoolchildren with asthma — estimates have run as high as 10 percent — and the roughly 50 percent higher absentee rate for asthmatic (as compared with nonasthmatic) children, an aggressive educational program to systematically bring together these youngsters would benefit not only the children but the school as well. Such a program, using American Lung Association materials, could be run by the school nurse, through the counseling office, or even by qualified volunteer personnel in the community. Additional self-management training materials are available through a variety of sources. The National Asthma Education Program provides a resource book titled *Managing Asthma: A Guide for Schools*, which contains a model plan for serving students with asthma. Asthmatic children should be able to participate in all school activities. (See Appendix I.)

The ALA has developed a series of age-related programs designed to teach elementary school children about care of the lungs. It is possible for schools to secure these materials from their local Lung and Heart Associations and to incorporate them in the school's general health education program.

Community-Based Groups

Community-based educational or support programs have been attempted in a number of places, primarily under the auspices of local chapters of the American Lung Association. One serious drawback to the effective use of these programs is the tendency to participate only in time of crisis — when the stress generated by the disease becomes acute. Without a crisis brewing there is unfortunately little incentive and consequently little obvious reason to give up time, energy, and comfort to attend these sessions. Obviously the crisis-generated approach fails to capitalize on some of the real advantages that a rational program of prevention and preparedness provides. We heartily encourage you to search for such a program, to get it *in advance of need*, and to stay with it faithfully once enrolled. You will find the benefits worth the effort.

In addition to local programs, three national asthma training programs for children have been developed. *Superstuff,* a self-training program for children, is designed to give parents and elementary school children more self-confidence, self-control, and know-how in dealing with their asthma. It does this by having the child work through a series of games, puzzles, and other exercises aimed at training the youngster to react appropriately to various aspects of the disease. The attractive workbook which is the core of this program can be purchased from your local American Lung Association office, which developed and sponsors this program.

ACT (Asthma Care Training) *for Kids* is supported by the Asthma and Allergy Foundation. Your local allergy society will know the location of the program, which consists of five one-hour sessions aimed at asthmatic children aged 6 to 12 and their parents. It is usually offered to small groups in which it tries to develop mastery skills and provide practice in decision-making for the child. Parents are taught how to nurture the child and create an environment conducive to decision-making.

Winning Over Wheezing is an asthma self-help program offered to children from 5 to 16 and their parents. It aims to improve knowledge about the disease, provides training in breathing and relaxation, and fosters self-management. It also stresses physical fitness; exercise (swimming is favored) is an integral part of every one of the 11 weekly sessions. The program is offered through the local pediatric society, which will know of the existence of any current or projected courses.

There are five other formal asthma training programs for children that may be offered in your community: *Open Airways*/Respiro Abierto, *Living with Asthma, Air Power, Air Wise,* and *C.A.L.M. (Child Asthmatics Learning to*

Manage Signals). Development of the first four programs has been supported by the National Heart, Lung, and Blood Institute, and may be sponsored locally by private medical practices, hospitals, clinics, American Lung Association affiliates, health maintenance organizations, and schools. The target groups, teaching techniques, curricula, and objectives sought vary from one program to another. Your local ALA branch will know of and be able to direct you to any of these programs that are being offered. Materials about *C.A.L.M.* are distributed by CIGNA Health Plan. (See Appendix I for the addresses of several self-management programs.)

In some communities local interest groups have been formed. These groups hold regular meetings, discussions, and (sometimes) a telephone hot line network. These interest groups are effective in disseminating information and are particularly valuable in teaching parents and children how to manage the psychological complications of asthma, notably the fear and helplessness that so often accompany it.

Enrolling in community-based programs is worth the effort involved in seeking them out. Get in touch with your local American Lung Association chapter. They will know if there are any local programs going on in your community. In addition, check with the allergy department of your local hospital, or the local chapter of the Asthma and Allergy Foundation (call the local medical society to find out the one nearest you) or pediatric society for information about community training and self-management programs. (See Appendix G for additional information.)

LONG-TERM RESIDENTIAL CARE FACILITIES

There are many institutions in the United States that offer long-term care for asthmatic children. These institutions cater to children who have "intractable" asthma; that is, asthma that does not respond to ordinary (or even extraordinary) medical measures.

An important element in the successful treatment of many of these severely ill children seems to be the reduction of family stress, a significant component of, or complication in, their asthma. In some cases dramatic improvement in symptoms has been noted on admission and separation from family without heroic medical attention. Taking the child out of a stressful environment evidently has the effect of eliminating the triggers and greatly reducing the severity of the symptoms.

Long-term residential care usually entails a broadly gauged multidisciplinary treatment approach that employs early and aggressive medical intervention and invokes self-management programs with some reliance on behavior modification training techniques. Psychological/psychiatric intervention with the child and the family may also represent an important part of the treatment.

171
SUMMER CAMPS
AND OTHER
SPECIAL
TREATMENT AND
CARE PROGRAMS

Daily costs run from nothing to over $200 per day, with costs being shared by state, institution, and individual (which includes health insurance). Length of stay may run from days to years, with the average treatment time running about six months. All of the institutions provide some schooling, and most can accommodate children from preschool through secondary school. Most of them will accept patients from out of state.

The principal objective of the long-term treatment facility is to bring the child to the point where asthma ceases to be the focal point of existence and to open up the possibility of leading a normal life. Resolution of psychological issues, attainment of effective control of symptoms, and individual assumption of responsibility for self-management are important subsidiary goals.

While long-term residential care is appropriate in some instances, it has its drawbacks. The regional nature of the hospitals causes logistical problems in some families, and it is often difficult to find a place because of the shortage of beds.

Where long-term care is not possible, one interesting recent development has been the establishment of short-term intensive care programs in a few centers. These programs, which embody most of the elements found in the longer-term counterparts, offer a useful community-based alternative and enjoy marked success in returning children to home and community in a relatively brief (two months on the average) period of time.

To locate either long- or short-term care facilities, consult the *Asthma Recovery Directory* referred to in Appendix H, or call any of the organizations listed in Appendix G, beginning with your local Lung Association.

Traveling with Asthma

GENERAL PRECAUTIONS

The most important thing to remember while traveling is to carry a supply of your medication or drugs sufficient to see you through the entire trip and to have them in a place where you can get to them *immediately* if you need them. Make it a point always to stow your medications in your carry-on luggage, and don't leave home without them. If you are sensitive to perfume, for example, and the only seat you can get on an airplane is next to a passenger who reeks of musk or lavender, having your Alupent inhaler buried in your suitcase in the baggage compartment will not help you much. Nor will it help you if you are bound for London and your luggage containing medication winds up in Karachi. (If you are assigned to the smoking section where you should not and do not want to be, don't hesitate to ask the flight attendant to help you make a seat change.)

Some recent evidence reveals that airplane travel may be especially dangerous for asthmatics, since the airline companies have been systematically cutting back on the supply of conditioned air in order to reduce their fuel costs. Be alert to this possibility. If it becomes necessary, complain and ask for full operation of the air conditioning equipment. This is particularly true when the plane is parked on the runway or is being held at the gate.

If there is a possibility that you may require emergency treatment for your asthma, be sure that you are wearing a Medic-Alert bracelet and have a statement as to what could cause a severe reaction in you and how it ought to be handled. Your physician can provide you with a letter carrying this information. Keep it in your billfold or passport.

SPECIFIC TIPS

You already realize that the surest way to prevent asthmatic episodes is to know and avoid whatever it is that provokes them. While this is tricky enough ordinarily, it can represent even more of a problem for the traveling asthmatic. You can circumvent it, though, by carefully relating the *cause* of your asthma to the *when, where,* and *how* of your trip. While we cannot anticipate every situation every asthmatic is likely to face, an example or two will give you the feeling of what we mean and help you to develop your own plan for steering around most of the potential trouble spots.

> Robert has severe asthmatic reactions to pollens, especially ragweed *(CAUSE)*. He wants to fly *(HOW)* to his sister Margaret's wedding, which is to be held in Iowa City *(WHERE)* on August 20 *(WHEN)*. He wants to decide if he should attend or not.

For the asthmatic traveler who is susceptible to pollens, the first thing to find out is what the pollen situation will be like at the destination or destinations. For travel in the United States or Canada you can determine in advance what pollen conditions are going to be like at any time of the year. The most easily accessible source is *The Manual of Allergy and Immunology* edited by Drs. Glenn Lawlor and Thomas Fischer and published by Little, Brown and Company. Robert's allergist doubtless owns a copy as would hospital or medical school libraries. Drug companies have also collected such information and extremely useful pollen guides are available on request from Hollister-Stier or Center Laboratories.* All of these references agree that ragweed pollen production would be at its peak in Iowa during August and September. By seeking out these references and knowing what to expect, Robert can make his decision and what precautions he ought to take in the form of preventive medication, housing, and so on. In Robert's case, flying is probably the best way to go because travel by automobile through ragweed country at the height of the pollen season would undoubtedly cause him considerable distress — even with the windows up and the air conditioning going full.blast.

Statistics about airborne allergens other than pollen which trigger asthmatic attacks have not been compiled, although it is easily possible to ascertain what the air quality is likely to be in major U.S. cities by consulting the weather page of a large daily newspaper published in the area you intend to visit. If smog triggers an asthmatic reaction for you and you have to make a trip to Denver in June, call your local weather service for information or ask your local library to get you a microfilm of the *Denver Post* for June a year ago. When it arrives, look up the air quality statistics for the period and, based on your knowledge or your reaction to polluted

---

* *Pollen Guide for Allergy*, Hollister-Stier, P.O. Box 3145, T.A., Spokane, WA 99220; *Pollen Aeroallergens of the United States*, Center Laboratories, 35 Channel Drive, Port Washington, NY 11050.

air, decide about the wisdom of a trip to the Mile High City at that time. If you cannot put off the trip and June is bad for smog in Denver, carry appropriate medication and observe the other precautions we spell out in Chapter 6. Also bear in mind that air pollution readings — "low," "moderate," etc. — relate to ordinary, nonasthmatic people. A low reading may affect a person with asthma more drastically than moderate pollution affects someone without asthma.

> Celeste is excited about her tour of the East African game parks. She will fly *(HOW)* to Nairobi, Kenya *(WHERE)* in July *(WHEN)*. She expects to have a marvelous time, but she is a little worried about accidentally consuming tartrazine (yellow food dye) *(CAUSE)*, which always triggers a serious asthmatic reaction in her.

Celeste will have to watch her step all along the way. She is likely to run into tartrazine in the airline food and in other processed foods she will be exposed to in Africa and any other continents en route. Worse, the requirements about package labeling of contents are not as stiff in many other countries as they are in the United States, and the contents, if named at all, will be listed in the language of the country. Celeste can try to stay away from preserved or processed foods entirely when she is out of the country. She should also let the tour director know of her problem in advance so that he or she is alert to the problem and can help Celeste find safe things to eat and knows of the possibility of a severe reaction in the event of a slip-up. Tours usually provide some variety in food choices, so Celeste should be quite safe as long as she keeps alert and takes no chances.

If you are going to a part of the world where the food is radically different from what you usually eat, and you react asthmatically to some foods, identify everything you are about to consume. Check it against a food family chart. (See Appendix E.) If what you are about to eat is a member of the same family of foods that cause you to wheeze, put it aside no matter how good it looks.

For the other major causes of asthma — vigorous exercise, exposure to extreme cold, and upper respiratory infections — following the same precautions you do at home, and faithfully keeping up with exercises and medication, should see you through. If you do react severely to extreme cold or low humidity, you should consider choosing a travel or vacation site that is compatible with your condition. Swimming in Barbados would be considerably less troublesome than trekking in the Himalayas.

Sleeping in New or Different Quarters

If you have intrinsic asthma, new environments and strange rooms will make little or no difference in your breathing or respiratory problems. On the other hand, if you have extrinsic asthma due to mold, animal dander, or dust, new rooms and new beds pose special problems.

Susan is extremely sensitive to house dust and animal dander. While on a trip she stopped at a motel. The motel and the room looked clean enough, but Susan began to wheeze severely almost as soon as she entered the room. It did not take her long to figure out that some previous occupants had brought their pet cat into the room with them. Susan had already paid the night's fee but was smart enough to realize she was in trouble. She packed her bags and went to a motel that did not allow pets. By explaining the problem she even got her room fee back.

Other problems with hotels, inns, and motels include the fact that many have musty, moldy odors from multiple years of use and abuse and worn carpets that retain dander and dust. Before you consider bedding down for the night, inspect the room carefully before you pay and consider the following:

- Does the room smell moldy or musty?
- Is there dust on the surfaces? In the corners? Under the furniture?
- Were animals previously permitted to reside in the room?
- Does it smell of cigarette or other tobacco smoke?

If the answer to any of these is yes, and if your asthma is exacerbated by any of them, move on.

Allergy Shots While Traveling

Patients who receive allergy injections need not be tied to a rigorous schedule of shots given at certain hours on given days. Allergy shots can safely be missed for several weeks, particularly when you have been on maintenance therapy for some time. As pointed out in Chapter 17, it is extremely important that you not administer the shot yourself. The shot should be administered by a doctor or nurse in an environment where emergency equipment is available, in case of a serious allergic or anaphylactic reaction. Accordingly, if you plan to be gone for an extended period of time, and if you want to continue taking your allergy shots during this period, carry a vial of the shot preparation with you. In addition, do the following:

- Have your doctor prepare written instructions on when and how much of the shot should be administered. Ask her or him to list what is in the vial and to label it. No doctor will inject vaccine from an unlabeled vial.
- Keep the vial refrigerated. Pack it in a styrofoam ice chest, or ask the desk clerk at the motel or hotel to refrigerate it for you.

If you are going to be in one location for a length of time, don't worry about carrying the allergy shot with you while traveling. Simply arrange for your doctor to ship it to your away-from-home address.

Travel and Medication

Traveling with medication generally poses no problems. The pills or capsules and the metered aerosols take little space and can be carried in purse or hand luggage where they are immediately available in case of need. They can be taken easily and inconspicuously. However, if you use a DeVilbiss Pulmo-Aide or other similar air compressor delivery system, you may run into difficulties. This device, as we indicated in Chapter 15, is simply an air compressor that nebulizes and efficiently delivers cromolyn or beta agonists such as Alupent. These machines generally have to be plugged into an electric outlet to work, and this can pose a problem on long automobile trips. They cost approximately $165. It is inconvenient to have to stop the car and go into a restroom at a gas station to plug in the Pulmo-Aide. Besides, service station restrooms are often moldy and dirty so that the compressor merely sends dirty air into your or your child's lungs. DeVilbiss, as well as other companies, makes a device with an adapter that plugs into and works off of the car's cigarette lighter. It costs approximately $225, but many local respiratory societies help needy families with the purchase price. Some hospital and sickroom supply firms rent home air compressors. One model, the Travelmate, has the advantage of a rechargeable battery and can plug into either a wall socket or a car cigarette lighter. It costs approximately $450.

Airports and large bus stations generally have first-aid rooms with provisions to plug in such machines. The machines are small enough to be carried easily and will fit under your seat.

Travel to foreign countries may pose a problem. The electrical outlets and current are different from those in the U.S. If you plan on traveling abroad, take a supply of socket adapters and a small transformer that will convert the local current to 120 volts. These converters are available in several forms from large department stores or luggage stores.

Summer Camps

Asthma is a fairly common problem, and most summer camps that have been in business for a number of years have had experience in dealing with asthmatic children. If your child has mild or seasonal asthma, and wants to go to camp, you should send along medicine and discuss its use and your child's complaint beforehand with the camp physician. However, children with mild asthma still experience some new and different problems when they first attend camp.

• Arriving at camp generally means meeting new people. New people bring new germs. Germs bring colds, and colds make asthma worse.

- Camp housing is often in older, poorly ventilated, dusty, mold-ridden buildings.
- Exercise, a must in summer camp, often makes asthma worse because it is more strenuous or different from what your child is accustomed to.
- Children are embarrassed at having others see them take their medication, but if they miss their drugs their asthma may get worse.

By anticipating these problems you can make camp a happy experience for your child. It is important that you choose the camp according to the following criteria:

- Does the camp have immediate access to medical personnel?
- Does the camp have previous experience dealing with children with asthma?
- What is the environment like? Are the housing arrangements clean? Are there any obvious asthma-exacerbating factors like dust, mold, etc.?
- Is the child's counselor sensitive and concerned enough to spend any extra time that may be required to look out for your child?

There are many children with asthma who should not be sent off to summer camp. For them the new environment, the period away from home without close, immediate medical supervision, the moldy, dusty environment, and the strenuous exercise simply make camp impossible. There are, however, special camps geared entirely to children with respiratory problems. The features and advantages of these special camps for moderate to severe asthmatic children are presented in Chapter 18.

Home Remedies and Alternative Strategies in the Treatment of Asthma

Asthma's stubbornness and its capacity to disable its victims for varying periods of time understandably makes them prime candidates for experimentation with various treatments. The chronic asthmatic wants nothing so much as to be free of symptoms and is willing to try anything to achieve that freedom. This yearning makes the treatment of asthma attractive to unscrupulous operators who promote a variety of abstruse schemes and devices. In seeking help, be wary of what is being offered and who is offering it.

The approach to care that we have followed in this book is essentially a traditional medical one, although we strongly emphasize the importance and benefits of an informed and aggressive program of self-care. To be effective, such a program depends on the determination and the ability to act intelligently and knowledgeably in finding appropriate and congenial help. In earlier chapters we presented procedures to follow in finding the best resources for treatment and control of asthma. See also Appendix G for the names and addresses of national organizations and associations that will be helpful to you in your search for medical, educational, and self-care resources.

ALTERNATIVE NONMEDICAL TREATMENT OPTIONS

If you or your child is a moderate to severe chronic asthmatic, any or all of the alternative nonmedical treatment options may attract you. These alternatives are likely to be mentioned or discussed in a number of places such as the classified advertisements in counterculture magazines; uncritical or undocumented accounts of "cures" appearing in the popular media; reports by family, friends, or neighbors who have heard of the treatment, who know somebody who benefited from it, or who themselves attest to its efficacy in their own case; or, most recently, radio and TV programs that feature lay health commentators who are eager to report a "medical breakthrough" no matter how fragmentary or tentative the evidence behind it may be. Anyone who has had to endure the pain, the discomfort, and the feeling of helplessness brought on by persistent asthma is likely to be intrigued by — and tempted to try — any remedy that seems to offer quick, complete relief. We believe, however, that these alternative strategies for the treatment of asthma are not as effective or time-efficient as conventional medical treatment. But we (and we hope your own personal physician) respect your right to choose and would view sympathetically your search for alternative therapies. We would also hope to remain informed of what you are doing and to provide medical advice and treatment when appropriate or requested. Although any of these treatments may bring some relief of symptoms, these remedies most often do not provide genuine, sustained relief. In some cases they actually make matters worse by diverting individuals away from appropriate treatment measures.

The major alternative approaches to treatment of asthma are

- Acupuncture
- Herbalism
- Homeopathy
- Naturopathy
- Osteopathy and chiropractic

Alternative treatments differ from conventional forms of medical treatment in two important ways. First, alternative approaches assume that what is wrong with the individual can be traced to something systemically wrong with the body. Their practitioners are more apt to consider disease entities as the result of a breakdown of bodily defenses; conventional medical thought, on the other hand, is inclined to regard bodily breakdown as effect rather than cause. The nontraditional view is not completely at odds with current medical thought and practice but mainly represents a difference in emphasis.

Second, alternative approaches derive from a different set of assumptions about the nature and workings of the body. Conventional medical thought grows out of the Western scientific view, which is inclined to emphasize precise diagnosis and equally narrow treatment efforts.

Ed hardly recognized Maurice, who had wasted away, gone completely gray, had lost most of his hair, and was obviously under chemical treatment for cancer. They had lunch together. Maurice indicated that he had just come from his biweekly treatment at the acupuncturist's. "Is it helping?" Ed asked. "I believe in it, so it helps," Maurice replied. He died two months later.

Maurice's case illustrates an important point about traditional medical and alternative therapies. The acupuncture did not cure him, but conventional chemical treatment had not been effective either. The alternative therapy did provide reassurance, relief of pain, and a source of support that proved comforting.

181
HOME REMEDIES
AND ALTERNATIVE
STRATEGIES IN THE
TREATMENT OF
ASTHMA

Acupuncture

Acupuncture (which has many variations) proceeds from the premise that disease is the result of an imbalance in the "energies" that course or flow throughout the body. This imbalance, for example, is said to permit bacteria to proliferate. By inserting long, slender needles (or by administering minute electrical charges or medication through needles; or by using acupressure, which does not require needles at all) at various points along the energy paths ("meridians"), the practitioner is able to normalize or stabilize the energy flow, and health is restored.

Acupuncture has enjoyed something of a vogue in the United States in the past 20 years. It has had considerable acceptance by physicians who use it to treat migraine, psoriasis, osteoarthritis, and joint pain, among other complaints, and pain relief generally. It does apparently relieve the pain associated with a number of chronic conditions.

Some acupuncture procedures are recommended for the treatment of asthma. Furthermore, there is scientific evidence to indicate that, when administered properly, it is associated with modest improvement in respiratory flow, decreased need for medication, and decline in subjective reports of symptoms.

Herbalism

Herbalism is certainly a companion to, and has been an important element in, medicine for thousands of years. It is still followed by those who believe in the efficacy and the essential conservatism of the method. Indeed, many medications still in favor and use grow out of the herbal tradition, and there is a recent, renewed interest in discovering the ability of herbs to affect body processes. For example, cromolyn was originally found in a weed.

Herbalists are likely to take a very detailed history. They then usually outline a program of diet, exercise, and herbal treatment aimed to improve your health status. Underlying the treatment is a whole-body approach, based on the view that the body is an aggregation of systems, some of which (according to the symptoms) may need toning or cleansing if health is to be restored. Thus, in addition to herbal remedies, dietary and stress-reducing measures might be recommended.

Coupled with the more general systemic treatments, there are a large number of herbs (herbs are defined as plants used as medicines) that are said to relieve asthmatic symptoms. Teas made of mullein, elecampane, ephedra, eucalyptus, horehound, lungwort, and pleurisy root are recommended to ease asthmatic coughing and to raise mucus; so is an infusion of garlic, ground ivy, blackthorn, and blue vervain; yerba santa mixed with cayenne, gum plant, vervain, and blackthorn and simmered in water is said to relieve bronchospasms.

These herbs are listed in standard medical references as treatments for asthma; the fact that they are not relied on to any great extent nowadays is because they are nowhere near as swift and powerful in their effect as the medications that have come to supplant them. Herbalists acknowledge this readily and contend that although herbal procedures take time, they are more effective in the long run in that they strengthen the body's natural tendency to seek health.

Serious herbalistic treatment with adequate follow-through might be expected to result in some reduction in the frequency and severity of asthmatic symptoms, but neither it nor conventional medicine is capable of overcoming the underlying genetic and physiological disposition to the disease.

Occasionally we are asked about the use of marijuana for asthma. Besides being illegal, there is no evidence that it is of any value. Moreover, marijuana is extremely irritating to the airways and the lungs. We strongly advise everyone (and especially asthmatics) to avoid it!

Homeopathy

Homeopathy is a "natural" system of healing or therapeutic method. It is based on the premise that a remedy can cure a disease only if it is capable of triggering symptoms similar to that of the disease in a well individual. Established by Samuel Hahnemann, a German physician, in the early part of the last century, it advances a law and set of postulates that provide a guide to treatment. Whereas the system and the arguments for it are much too elaborate to be repeated here, the essential philosophy can be summarized as follows:

- Any pharmacologically active substance can cause symptoms to appear in a healthy individual, and these symptoms are characteristic of that substance.
- Anyone suffering from any disease shows a set of symptoms that are characteristic of the disease.
- A cure (the disappearance of symptoms) may be obtained by administering the substance whose symptoms *exactly* match those presented by the disease.

This is analogous to what happens in the process of desensitization through the administration of allergy shots. The ill person takes extremely dilute solutions of the substance, which produces the symptoms that match those produced by the disease. The result is immunity and loss of symptoms. If the symptoms do not vanish, try again until you find the one substance that perfectly matches the symptoms.

Certainly, some elements of homeopathic thought do appear in traditional medical practice, and, as we have noted, immunization and desensitization rest on what Hahnemann advanced as homeopathic principles. To a limited extent it is useful as a concept, but in practice the method is so highly individualized, arcane, and slow that it is of little or no value in the treatment of anything but the mildest type of asthma symptoms. Apart from that, we have already indicated that desensitization, insofar as asthma is concerned, is rarely appropriate and carries with it substantial risks. Finally, homeopathy seems to assume that all diseases are unitary and that any "interconnectedness" (of allergic complaints, for example, where symptoms may be extremely diffuse and in conflict with one another when it comes to treatment) would pose a difficult therapeutic decision.

Naturopathy

Naturopathy is a very old belief system whose keystone is the mechanism of homeostasis — the tendency of the body to seek and maintain a state of equilibrium, or balance.

Naturopaths (who are not recognized as medical specialists in the United States) are apt to refer to themselves as holistic healers whose efforts are directed at people rather than at ailments. In practice they regard each person as unique, having a constellation of capabilities, characteristics, and needs different from those displayed by any other person.

The naturopath tries, through history and observation in a variety of modes and levels, to discover this whole, unique individual and to establish the underlying causes of illness.

Once established, treatment is directed at eradicating causes rather than attacking symptoms; treatment itself may utilize some combination of herbalism, homeopathy, massage, psychological counseling, acupuncture, biofeedback, or any of a variety of other approaches.

We believe that, while naturopathy is based on some fundamentally sound principles, such discovery and treatment of the unique, many-faceted individual represents a task beyond the present capability of any specialty or specialist.

Osteopathy and Chiropractic

These two specializations differ greatly in the amount of training required for certification. In many states osteopaths are accepted as coequal with physicians and practice on an equal footing with them.

Chiropractors must have a state-issued license, but their training period is considerably shorter and narrower than that for osteopaths or physicians. Physicians generally dismiss the assumption that certain kinds of mechanical adjustments to the body (especially of subluxations or misalignments of vertebrae in the spinal column) can bring about improvement in asthma; osteopaths and chiropractors hold to this viewpoint in varying degrees.

Not all chiropractors will try to treat asthma. Many are now likely to be interested in the dietary and other habits of their patients and to recommend a broadly based, "holistic" treatment regimen.

Nevertheless, most physicians contend that strict chiropractic or osteopathic treatment of asthma is futile. Certainly there is no persuasive scientific evidence indicating that chiropractic treatment of asthmatics has led to the easing or remission of their symptoms, and there is no obvious reason to believe that the manipulations and adjustments that are an integral part of this sort of therapy would have any effect either on the agents that cause asthmatic reactions or on the bronchospasms that are the result of the asthmatic's twitchy airways. Despite this, many clinical reports of chiropractic success with asthma do exist. These may have occurred possibly because of the relief of underlying psychological stress or tension that contributed to the bronchospasms and the resulting symptoms.

NONTRADITIONAL METHODS OF TESTING AND TREATMENT

The history of medicine is filled with examples of treatments that enjoyed great popularity for a time until they were found to be ineffectual or to have even made symptoms worse. Asthma has had its share of dubious treatments over the years, and there are three treatment strategies currently in vogue that claim to be able to determine nutritional deficiencies: hair analysis, cytotoxic testing, and Candida testing. A fourth general approach to asthma is clinical ecology.

Hair Analysis

Hair analysis may be recommended to measure your nutritional status. Hair analysis is a very precise, accurate procedure when done *correctly*. A properly conducted hair analysis would first have you wash your hair completely and not put any hair preparations on it until the test is complete. Next, an area on your scalp would be shaved and new hair allowed to grow for the next few weeks. It is this new, never-been-washed hair that is analyzed. Otherwise, all you are analyzing is the chemical composition of your shampoo or hair spray.

> Pete has suffered with "tension fatigue" for many years. Both a doctor and a few sessions with a psychologist did not resolve his problem. He read an article on hair analysis and sent a sample of his hair off to be studied, hoping it would reveal the cause.
>   The analysis cost Pete $50 and showed that he had a tremendous amount of zinc in his hair — 100 times the amount of zinc that he should have had. Pete was both elated and depressed at these results. He was elated because something wrong was found and depressed because he did not know what to do. He read that zinc was in meat as well as in many other things. He put himself on a

drastic program, eliminating all sources of zinc in his diet. He grew weak, lost weight, and, in time, his hair began to fall out. He went to see his doctor, who examined him, heard about the diet, and correctly concluded that Pete was now zinc deficient, a serious problem.

Pete insisted that he was not deficient but that he had too much zinc. He explained about the hair analysis. The doctor was not an expert on hair analysis and knew virtually nothing about it. He called a nutrition expert at a local university and presented the problem. The professor told the doctor to look at Pete's hair shampoo. Pete brought it in and found out it contained a heavy concentration of zinc oxide.

Nutritional deficiency has not been established as a cause of asthma. However, many people do have legitimate problems with nutrition. They may suffer from diabetes, intestinal disorders, or may even have a rare genetic disease that prevents normal metabolism. If those individuals also have allergies — including asthma — they should consult their physician and, if necessary, refer themselves to somebody skilled in clinical nutrition. Be sure that the nutritionist has had formal training in a nutrition department in a university medical school. Unhappily, there is no board certification in nutrition, so anybody can hang up a shingle as a clinical nutritionist. It is up to you to check their credentials. The best place to start your search for a qualified nutritionist is at a local university or your county medical society. Unfortunately, people who advocate hair analysis are likely to have vested financial interests in the laboratories that do hair analyses and therefore have something to gain from ordering them.

Cytotoxic Testing

Cytotoxic testing is likely to be done by a physician who is interested in or claims to practice something called "ecological" or "orthomolecular" medicine. This practitioner believes that your asthma symptoms are most likely linked to your reactions to different foods or chemicals and will have you undergo a series of tests to identify what it is that is causing your asthma. In this form of testing, the white cells are removed from a sample of your blood. Then the cells are mixed with extracts of foods or chemicals believed to be responsible for your symptoms, and the mixture is studied under a microscope. If the white cells seem to be dead, you are said to be allergic to whatever has been mixed with the cells.

This is an attractive and superficially plausible procedure, but it has one basic shortcoming: *it does not work*. Recent laboratory studies have compared individuals known to be free of allergies with people with known allergies. Cytotoxic testing failed to differentiate between the two groups and did not identify the specific allergens reliably.

Cytotoxic testing has been judged to be useless by the Food and Drug Administration and by the American Academy of Allergy and Immunology. California physicians using cytotoxic testing are being sued by the state's Board of Medical Quality Assurance for, among other things, fraudulent advertising, unfair business practices, and conspiracy to violate the state's Business and Professions code. If a physician or other health practitioner recommends that you undergo cytotoxic testing, seek other help.

Candida

There have been a number of reports circulated of people suffering from weakness, tension fatigue, and even occasionally mild to moderate asthma who are said to have Candida or Monilia (yeast) infections throughout their body. The reports contend that these infections are occult, not revealed by conventional methods of detection. Nonetheless, it is believed that a yeast infection is present in the body and releases certain products, including alcohol, which bring about personality change and produce a wide variety of symptoms, including allergic ones. The reports go on to claim that, when these people are treated with antifungal antibiotics, they often get better.

The Candida connection to asthma is even more flimsy than some of the alternative therapies we have already discussed. If you did have Monilia or Candida in your body, you would almost certainly be gravely ill. Your body simply cannot tolerate fungal infections beneath the skin. Whereas you may get yeast infections in your intestinal tract, mouth, or vagina, these areas are all considered to be external. To suggest that Candida infections inside the body are producing these infections is absurd; to treat it with broad spectrum antibiotics is not only pointless but may cause unnecessary and potentially harmful side effects.

Clinical Ecology

Clinical ecology is not an established medical specialty like orthopedics or dermatology. It is simply an outlook or an approach to the practice of medicine, particularly the treatment of individuals who are troubled by generalized stress-fatigue symptoms or allergic-like reactions, including asthma.

The assumption behind clinical ecology is that these reactions and the fatigue-stress symptoms are the result of subtle and insidious effects of any of a multiplicity of possible causal factors. To these practitioners much of what ails people — from itchiness to madness to obesity — is traceable to allergic or hypersensitive reactions to something in the environment. Foods are saddled with much of the blame, but synthetics, chemicals, plastics, and emissions come in for their share of criticism.

To the clinical ecologist there is no such thing as intrinsic asthma — everything is extrinsic; i.e., has a cause somewhere in the environment which can be located if one looks hard and long enough. This is an attractive notion, but the search for the ecological villain may be long, expensive, and, in the end, futile. Sometimes the therapeutic strategy will be the preparation of an ecologically "pure" environment, which can use up a good deal of your cash and achieve no more than much simpler avoidance tactics supplemented by an appropriate and judicious course of medication that anticipates and controls your asthma symptoms.

A second problem with clinical ecology is that, whereas its practitioners are messianic in their zeal, and there are many individuals around who attest fervently to what, in retrospect, seems to be their near-miraculous cures, there is no persuasive evidence to bear out the contention that many of the vague, annoying, debilitating symptoms are the result of allergies or hypersensitivity to anything. We have no quarrel with advice to eat sensibly and to live in an environment that is as free of contamination as it is possible to make it. When carried to extremes, however — and this often seems to be the case with clinical ecology — it is an overwhelming and ultimately limiting outlook.

A Note about Vitamins

There are some people who claim that asthmatics have some genetic or familial abnormality in body metabolism that leads to vitamin or mineral deficiencies or abnormalities in sugar metabolism. The evidence for this abnormality is very weak, although there is no doubt at all that adequate nutrition is vital for good health. However, this does not mean that suboptimal nutrition will result in asthma or allergies.

We discussed earlier in this book the necessity for a good, sound diet, one likely to give your body the nutrients and minerals it needs. We believe that the actual recommended daily allowances for many vitamins and minerals may not always be sufficient for asthmatics. These recommended daily allowances are based on limited observations and often do not take into account the additional stresses and needs brought on by chronic illness, by interactions of diet with medications you are using, and by possible changes in requirements as you get older. For this reason we unhesitatingly recommend the use of a good multivitamin preparation, should you have any doubts at all about the adequacy of your diet. It does not have to be expensive. It should contain all of the B vitamins and vitamin C as well as minerals including zinc. Table 16 lists what we think should be in your multivitamin or family vitamin. These vitamins, incidentally, are generic and can be bought over-the-counter. They are identical to and much less expensive than heavily advertised, brand-name vitamins.

TABLE 16   Essentials of a Good Multivitamin

Vitamin A	Folic Acid
Vitamin B1 (Thiamine)	Iron
Vitamin B2 (Riboflavin)	Niacinamide
Vitamin B6 (Pyridoxine)	Pantothenic Acid
Vitamin B12	Vitamin E
Vitamin C	Zinc

Appendix A: Elimination Diet for Asthma

Follow this elimination diet *only* with the knowledge of, and after consultation with, your physician.

Foods Allowed

Beverages
Water

Dessert
Tapioca

*Fruits and Juices
Apricots
Cranberries
Peaches
Pears

Grains and Cereals
Rice
Rice flakes, Rice Krispies
Puffed Rice
Rice wafers

Meats
Lamb

Oils
Crisco, Spry
Olive oil
Any vegetable oil *except* oleomargarine

Seasonings
Acetic acid vinegar (white)
Salt
Vanilla extract (synthetic)

Sweeteners
Sugar (cane or beet)

*Vegetables
Beets
Carrots
Chard
Lettuce
Oyster plant
Sweet potato

*All fruits and vegetables, except lettuce, must be cooked or canned.

Eat and Drink *Only* the Foods Listed

AVOID: Coffee, tea, soft drinks, chewing gum, all medications except those ordered by your doctor

Suggested Menu:

Breakfast	*Lunch*	*Dinner*
Rice Krispies	Lamb chop	Lamb pattie
Rice wafers	Sweet potato	Boiled rice
Peaches	Beets	Carrots
Apricot juice	Rice wafers	Lettuce with acetic acid
Peach jam	Cranberry juice	Peaches
Water	Pears	Apricot juice

INSTRUCTIONS: Stay on this basic diet for 10 days. Then on the 11th day add, all by itself, first thing in the morning, the one food you believe is most likely responsible for your asthma symptoms. Eat in large amounts several times a day for three days and keep track of your reaction. If a reaction (wheezing, cough, shortness of breath) occurs, *stop*. Return to basic diet and after five days try again. If reaction reappears, avoid this food henceforth. Go on to test other foods suspected of causing symptoms in this same way. Foods not causing asthma symptoms may be retained in the diet.

Appendix B:
Foods Containing
Tartrazine

Tartrazine is a dye (FD&C yellow #5) added to foods to "improve" their appearance. The list below is only suggestive of the literally thousands of places it may turn up. Read labels carefully. A typical label may read as follows:

"INGREDIENTS: Enriched wheat flour . . . whole wheat flour . . . oil shortening . . . sugar, corn syrup, salt, malted barley flour, lecithin, *FD&C yellow #5*, and artificial color."

Baked goods, breads with food
   dyes added, sweet breads, whole
   wheat
Butter
Candies
Cereals, colored
Cheeses
Chips (potato, corn, taco)
Fish, frozen (some; check label)
Fruits, canned (some; check label)
Ice creams

Jello (gelatin)
Lozenges
Margarine
Meats, prepared
Mouthwash
Mustard
Pudding
Sauces and gravies, prepared
Toothpaste
Yogurt

Appendix C:
Foods Containing
Metabisulfite

Metabisulfite (sodium bisulfite) is a food preservative and freshener. Although its use has been regulated by the Food and Drug Administration, the regulations are haphazard to the point of being irrational. For example, one bunch in four of sulfited fresh table grapes must be tagged with a label stating that sulfite has been added. This encourages consumers to believe that the untagged clusters do *not* contain the chemical. In addition, imported preserved foods (Knorr soups, for instance) may contain sulfites that the overseas manufacturer is not required to list among the ingredients named on the package. Salad bars are probably safer than they were five years ago; still, metabisulfite may turn up in many processed foods including beer and wine and may also be added, unannounced, to certain foods especially prone to spoilage. Foods likely to contain sulfite include:

Beer
Cheeses
Cider
Cordials
Fruit juices
Glucose (syrup and solid)
Jello (gelatin)
Pickles
Potatoes, whole, peeled, or sliced (raw)
Salsa
Sausages and sausage meat
Vegetables, dehydrated (especially peas)
Vinegar
Wines (red, white, or rosé)

Appendix D: Foods Containing Salicylate*

Salicylate, especially as it occurs in aspirin-based medications, is a common and potent cause of asthmatic symptoms. It is also employed as a preservative and appears in many foods including those listed below. A typical medication label reads as follows:

"INGREDIENTS: *Aspirin* 400 mg., caffeine 32 mg." (Aspirin is technically called acetylsalicylic acid.)

Beverages: Any alcoholic beverage, cider, diet drinks, Kool-aid, soft drinks

Breads: Raisin bread, sweet bread

Cereals: All cold cereals (*except* puffed wheat, puffed rice) and hot cereals

Desserts: Ice cream, cookies, pies, cakes, cake mixes, gelatins

Meat, Eggs, Cheese: Lunch meats, pasteurized spreads and cheeses, frankfurters

Potatoes and Rice: All *except* unprocessed potatoes and rice

Sweets: Chocolate, gum, candy, jam, jelly, marmalade

Vegetables: All *except* cucumbers, pickles, tomato

Fats and Oils: Margarine

Fruits: Apples, apricots, blackberries, cherries, currants, gooseberries, grapes, raisins, nectarines, oranges, peaches, plums, raspberries, strawberries

Juices: All *except* pineapple, grapefruit, cranberry, pear

Miscellaneous: Cloves, allspice, oil of wintergreen, licorice, tooth powder, mint flavors, lozenges, mouthwash, perfumes, aspirins or medicines containing aspirin (*i.e.,* Bufferin, Anacin, Excedrin, Alka-Seltzer, Empirin compound)

*Salicylates occurring naturally in the above foods may not have such serious effects as those found in medications.

Appendix E:
Food Families

Family	Members
APPLE	Apple, pear, quince
ASTER	Lettuce, chicory, endive, escarole, artichoke, dandelion, sunflower seeds
BEET	Beet, spinach, chard
BLUEBERRY	Blueberry, huckleberry, cranberry
BUCKWHEAT	Buckwheat, rhubarb, garden sorrel
CASHEW	Cashew, pistachio, mango
CHOCOLATE	Chocolate (cocoa), cola
CITRUS	Orange, lemon, grapefruit, lime, tangerine, kumquat, citron
FUNGUS	Mushroom, yeast
GINGER	Ginger, cardamom, turmeric
GOOSEBERRY	Currant, gooseberry
GRAINS	Wheat, corn, rice, oats, barley, rye. Also: wildrice, cane, millet sorghum, bamboo shoots
LAUREL	Avocado, cinnamon, bay leaves, sassafras
MALLOW	Cottonseed, okra
MELON	Watermelon, cucumber, cantaloupe, pumpkin, squash, other melons
MINT	Mint, peppermint, spearmint, thyme, sage, basil, savory, rosemary, catnip

MUSTARD	Mustard, turnip, radish, horseradish, watercress, cabbage, kraut, chinese cabbage, broccoli, cauliflower, brussels sprouts, collards, kale, kohlrabi, rutabaga
MYRTLE	Allspice, guava, clove pimiento (not the red pepper form of pimiento)
ONION	Onion, garlic, asparagus, chives, leeks, sarsaparilla
PALM	Coconut, date
PARSLEY	Carrot, parsnip, celery, parsley, celeriac, anise, dill, fennel, angelica, celery seed, cumin, coriander, caraway
PEA	Peanuts, peas (green, field, blackeyed), beans (navy, lima, pinto, string, soy, etc.), licorice, acacia, tragacanth
PLUM	Plum, cherry, peach, apricot, nectarine, almond
POTATO	Potato, tomato, eggplant, green pepper, red pepper, chili pepper, paprika, cayenne
ROSE	Strawberry, raspberry, blackberry, dewberry, loganberry, youngberry, boysenberry
WALNUT	English walnut, black walnut, pecan, hickory nut, butternut

Appendix F:
The Asthma IQ Test

The following test was prepared by the National Heart, Lung, and Blood Institute as part of the National Asthma Education Program. It is reproduced with the kind permission of the National Asthma Education Program and the U.S. Department of Health and Human Services.

Answer the twelve true-or-false questions. Then read the answers that follow and score yourself. If you correctly answer eleven or twelve questions, you know a lot about asthma. If you answer fewer than ten questions correctly, you should try to learn more about asthma.

	True	False
1. Asthma is a common disease among children and adults in the United States.	☐	☐
2. Asthma is an emotional or psychological illness.	☐	☐
3. The way that parents raise their children can cause asthma.	☐	☐
4. Asthma episodes may cause breathing problems, but these episodes are not really harmful or dangerous.	☐	☐
5. Asthma episodes usually occur suddenly without warning.	☐	☐
6. Many different things can bring on an asthma episode.	☐	☐
7. Asthma cannot be cured, but it can be controlled.	☐	☐

8. There are different types of medicine to control asthma. ☐ ☐

9. People with asthma have no way to monitor how well their lungs are functioning. ☐ ☐

10. Both children and adults can have asthma. ☐ ☐

11. Tobacco smoke can make an asthma episode worse. ☐ ☐

12. People with asthma should not exercise. ☐ ☐

Answers on the following page.

Answers to the Asthma IQ Test

1. **TRUE.** Asthma is a common disease among children and adults in the United States, and it is increasing. About 10 million people have asthma, of whom 3 million are under 18 years of age.

2. **FALSE.** Asthma is not an emotional or psychological disease, although strong emotions can sometimes make asthma worse. People with asthma have sensitive lungs that react to certain things, causing the airways to tighten, swell, and fill with mucus. The person then has trouble breathing and may cough and wheeze.

3. **FALSE.** The way parents raise their children does not cause asthma. It is not caused by a poor parent-child relationship or by being overprotective.

4. **FALSE.** Asthma episodes can be very harmful. People can get very sick and need hospitalization. Some people have died from asthma episodes. Frequent asthma episodes, even if they are mild, may cause people to stop being active and living normal lives.

5. **FALSE.** Sometimes an asthma episode may come on quite quickly. However, before a person has any wheezing or shortness of breath there are usually symptoms such as a cough, a scratchy throat, or tightness in the chest. Most patients learn to recognize these early symptoms and can take medicine to prevent a serious episode.

6. **TRUE.** For most people with asthma, an episode can start from many different "triggers." Some of these things are pollen from trees or grasses; molds or house dust; weather changes; strong odors; cigarette smoke; and certain foods. Other triggers include being upset; laughing or crying hard; having a cold or the flu; or being near furry or feathered animals. Each person with asthma has an individual set of asthma "triggers."

7. **TRUE.** There is no cure yet for asthma. However, asthma patients can control it to a large degree by:
   - Getting advice from a doctor who treats asthma patients
   - Learning to notice early signs of an asthma episode and to start treatment
   - Avoiding things that cause asthma episodes
   - Taking medicine just as the doctor says
   - Knowing when to get medical help

8. **TRUE.** Several types of medicines are available to control asthma. Some people with mild asthma need to take medication only when they have symptoms. But most people need to take medicine every day to prevent symptoms and also to take medicine when symptoms do occur. A doctor needs to decide the best type of medicine for each patient and how often it should be taken. Asthma patients and their doctors need to work together to manage the disease.

9. **FALSE.** People with asthma can monitor how well their lungs are functioning with a peak flow meter. This small device can be used at home, work, or school. The peak flow meter may show that the asthma is getting worse before the usual symptoms appear.

10. **TRUE.** Both children and adults can have asthma. Sometimes, but not always, symptoms will go away as children get older. However, many children continue to have asthma symptoms throughout adulthood. In some cases, symptoms of asthma are not recognized until a person is an adult.

11. **TRUE.** Smoke from cigarettes, cigars and pipes can bring on an asthma attack. Indoor smoky air from fireplaces and outdoor smog can make asthma worse. Some can also "set off" other triggers. Smokers should be asked not to smoke near someone with asthma. Moving to another room may help, but smoke travels from room to room. No smoking is best for everyone!

12. **FALSE.** Exercise is good for most people — with or without asthma. When asthma is under good control, people with asthma are able to play most sports. For people whose asthma is brought on by exercise, medicines can be taken before exercising to help avoid an episode. A number of Olympic medalists have asthma.

Appendix G: Organizations Concerned with Asthma

American Academy of Allergy and Immunology
611 East Well Street
Milwaukee, WI 53202
1-800-822-2762

American College of Allergy and Immunology
800 East Northwest Highway
Suite 1080
Palatine, IL 60067
1-800-842-7777

American Lung Association
See the white pages of the telephone directory for phone number and address of your local Lung Association

Asthma and Allergy Foundation of America
National Headquarters
1717 Massachusetts Avenue, NW
Suite 305
Washington, DC 20036
1-800-727-8462

National Allergy and Asthma Network/Mothers of Asthmatics
3554 Chain Bridge Road
Suite 200
Fairfax, VA 22030
1-800-878-4403

National Asthma Education Program Information Center
4733 Bethesda Avenue
Suite 350
Bethesda, MD 20814-4820
1-301-951-3260

National Jewish Center for Immunology and Respiratory Medicine
1400 Jackson Street
Denver, CO 80206
1-800-222-LUNG (222-5864)

Appendix H:
Sources of Products for
People with Asthma

The best starting points for information about suppliers of products for asthmatics are the yellow pages, the *Asthma Resources Directory*, and your physician or health plan.

Yellow Pages. Here are some telephone directory listings that you may find helpful in locating local suppliers of supplies:

Air Cleaning and Purifying Equipment
Air Conditioners
Air Conditioning Equipment and Systems — Repairing
Clean Rooms — Installation and Equipment
Dust and Fume Collecting Systems
Dust Control Materials
Health Appliances
Health and Diet Food Products — Retail
Hospital Equipment and Supplies
Safety Equipment

Asthma Resources Directory. This book provides valuable information on makes and models of equipment, names of suppliers, and asthma self-help programs, including summer camps for children. It also discusses a variety of other aspects of asthma care. The book is expensive, so you may want to look for it in your local Lung Association office, a public or university library, or your HMO or allergist's library.

The *Asthma Resources Directory* is available for $29 plus $3 shipping and handling from the National Allergy and Asthma Network/Mothers of Asthmatics (see Appendix G).

Physicians or HMOs. These offices may be able to suggest local sources of supply for materials or devices that they recommend.

We have listed below some of the devices and materials frequently sought by individuals with asthma and the names of a few of the companies that supply them. However, these mentions should not be taken as an endorsement of any firm, product, or service. We have observed that enterprises specializing in products or services for asthmatics tend to have short life spans. Therefore, these addresses cannot be taken as a comprehensive list of resources.

General Suppliers. Large mercantile chains (Montgomery Ward, Sears, J. C. Penney, etc.) carry some of the products that people affected by asthma may require. Specialized stores include:

Allergy Control Products
96 Danbury Road
Ridgefield, CT 05877
1-203-438-9580

The Allergy Store
P.O. Box 2555
Sebastopol, CA 95473
1-800-824-7163

The AL-R-G Shop
3411 Johnson Street
Hollywood, FL 33021
1-305-981-9182

Masks/Respirators

A. J. Masuen Company
P.O. Box 768
Elk Grove Village, IL 60009
1-800-831-0894

Mine Safety Appliance Co.
519 Niagara Street
Tonawanda, NY 14150
1-716-691-6922

Nebulizers

DeVilbiss Health Care Worldwide
P.O. Box 635
Somerset, PA 15501
1-814-443-4881

DURA Pharmaceuticals, Inc.
P.O. Box 28331
San Diego, CA 92128
1-619-450-6690

Peak Expiratory Flow Meters. For more about these devices, see pages 43 and 133. The following company markets two such devices, one for "standard" and one for "low-range" readings.

Aller/Guard
1645 Southwest 41st Street
Topeka, KS 66609-1250
1-800-234-0816

Vacuum Cleaners. Some manufacturers advertise that their vacuum cleaners are specifically designed to deal with house dust and dust mites. These units are expensive and unproven, however.

Nilfisk of America, Inc.
300 Technology Drive
Malvern, PA 19355
1-800-NILFISK

Sanyo
21350 Lassen Street
Chatsworth, CA 91311-2329
1-818-998-7322
(Sanyo has not responded to requests for detailed information about the performance of its vacuum cleaner.)

Appendix I:
Asthma Education Programs
for Children

Superstuff. Developed by the American Lung Association, this is an educational program for elementary school children with their parents. Contact the local Lung Association office listed in your telephone directory for more information.

The Lung Association office can also tell you if a local organization is offering any of the four asthma training programs supported by the National Heart, Lung, and Blood Institute: **Open Airways/*Respiro Abierto*, Living With Asthma, Air Power,** and **Air Wise.**

Asthma Care Training (ACT) for Kids. The Asthma and Allergy Foundation created this program, which provides five one-hour sessions for children ages 6 to 12 who have asthma and their parents. Contact a local allergy group, or see Appendix G for the address of the Asthma and Allergy Foundation.

Child Asthmatics Learning to Manage Signals (C.A.L.M.) For information, contact:

CIGNA Health Plan
2502 Rocky Point Road
Tampa, FL 33067
1-813-884-2400

Winning Over Wheezing. For children ages 5 to 16 and their parents, this asthma self-management program consists of 11 weekly sessions that involve exercise and education. It is usually offered through the local pediatric society. Materials come from Rorer Pharmaceuticals. Write:

William H. Rorer, Inc.
Fort Washington, PA 19034
1-215-628-6000

Managing Asthma: A Guide for Schools. This resource book, prepared by the U.S. Department of Health and Human Services and the U.S. Department of Education, provides school personnel with practical ways to help students with asthma participate fully in all school activities, including physical education. It contains a model Asthma Action Plan that unites physician, parents, and school personnel in a comprehensive approach to serving a student with asthma. *Managing Asthma* is NIH Publication No. 91-2650. Copies may be obtained from:

National Asthma Education Program Information Center
4733 Bethesda Avenue
Suite 530
Bethesda, MD 20814-4820
1-301-951-3260

Index